DISEASE AND
ECONOMIC
DEVELOPMENT

DISEASE AND ECONOMIC DEVELOPMENT

The Impact Of Parasitic Diseases
In St. Lucia

Burton A. Weisbrod

Ralph L. Andreano

Robert E. Baldwin

Erwin H. Epstein

Allen C. Kelley

with the assistance of
Thomas W. Helminiak

THE UNIVERSITY OF WISCONSIN PRESS

PUBLISHED 1973
THE UNIVERSITY OF WISCONSIN PRESS
BOX 1379, MADISON, WISCONSIN 53701

THE UNIVERSITY OF WISCONSIN PRESS, LTD.
70 GREAT RUSSELL STREET, LONDON

FOR LC CIP INFORMATION SEE THE COLOPHON

ISBN 0–299–06340–2

CONTENTS

TABLES

ILLUSTRATIONS

(Photographs of St. Lucia by Burton A. Weisbrod, Erwin H. Epstein, and Thomas W. Helminiak.)

Figures in the text

PREFACE

This study owes an enormous debt of thanks to The Rockefeller Foundation and, more particularly, to the director and associate director of the foundation's Humanities and Social Science Division, Drs. Joseph Black and Ralph K. Davidson, who, in 1966, saw the need for a study of the economic and social impact of the world's reputedly number one public health disease, schistosomiasis. With financial support from The Rockefeller Foundation, the present book was produced by our group of four economists—including persons with interests in economic development (Robert E. Baldwin), demography (Allen C. Kelley), public finance and human resources (Burton A. Weisbrod), and economic history (Ralph L. Andreano)—and one sociologist (Erwin H. Epstein) with interests in comparative education and especially relationships between cultures and school systems. We embarked on the study with the ambitious objectives of not only assessing the effects of one disease in one limited region (St. Lucia, West Indies), but also of developing an analytical approach that would be a useful guide to researchers who might examine the impacts of other diseases in other regions.

Each chapter in this book was read and commented upon by all the authors. It is, therefore, a joint effort. Yet each chapter was primarily the work of one or two persons, who should be identified: chapter 1—Weisbrod and Baldwin; chapter 2—Andreano and Baldwin; chapters 3 and 4—Andreano. Chapter 5 summarizes our empirical efforts: the natality and mortality investigations by Kelley (described in detail in Appendix B), the studies of schoolchildren's performances by Epstein and Weisbrod (described more fully in Appendix C), and the analyses of labor productivity carried out by Baldwin and Weisbrod (described more completely in Appendix D). Chapter 5 was prepared by the authors of these technical empirical studies, with the assistance of Felicity Skidmore. Chapters 6 and 7 were authored by Weisbrod, with the assistance of certain material by Epstein in chapter 6. In addition to the appendices referred to above, Appendix F was authored by Weisbrod and Thomas W. Helminiak, Appendix G by Baldwin and Weisbrod, and Appendix H by Helminiak.

The data on the productivity of labor at the Geest banana plantations analyzed here cover the period January 1966–December 1968. Recently, we have acquired new productivity data for the period January 1969– December 1971 for 289 Geest workers who were parasitologically tested during the field work in St. Lucia described in this volume. As we point out in chapter 6, it is plausible to hypothesize that the debilitating effects of schistosomiasis and the other four parasitic infections may develop only after some years, and that serious infection in St. Lucia may be of relatively recent vintage. The passage of time would therefore reveal more severe impacts of disease. In the months ahead we will investigate the relationship between (1) disease infection at the time of the studies reported here, and (2) productivity of those same workers at a later date. An extremely tentative and preliminary impression of our new data is that there may be some evidence of a lagged response of labor productivity to parasite infection, although only a small portion of the new data has been analyzed.

We are anxious to acknowledge those who have worked with us on this study. First, we want to thank Dr. Peter Jordan, director of The Rockefeller Foundation-supported Research and Control Department in St. Lucia. Without his continued cooperation and assistance in carrying out medical examinations, in providing various data about the prevalence of schistosomiasis and other parasitic diseases in St. Lucia, and in countless other ways, our entire effort would have been impossible.

During the first two years of the study, Thomas Helminiak, then a Ph.D. candidate in economics at the University of Wisconsin and now a Ph.D. and research associate in our Health Economics Research Center, supervised our extensive data-gathering activities in St. Lucia, during which a household survey was undertaken, medical tests arranged, work records obtained and matched with medical information, and potential sources of data investigated. His contribution in this administrative role was substantial, and, in addition, he commented painstakingly on earlier drafts of the full manuscript.

Continuing in the fine tradition of Helminiak, Clark R. Bloom succeeded to the position of "our man in St. Lucia," where he supervised the data-gathering efforts during their final stages. Still another Ph.D. candidate in economics, Peter Lundt, directed our laborious efforts to obtain labor-productivity data from the work records of St. Lucia's largest grower of bananas, the Geest Company. These records proved extremely valuable to our research, and so we also want to thank those at Geest who provided us with access to this and other information concerning productivity on their estates—Francis J. Carasco, J. B. Etherington (deceased), Abel Ghirawoo, and Miss Lucille Lorde. Among those employed in our field operations in St. Lucia were Peter Dalton, George Compton, Claudius Louis, and Roland Polius. Others who aided us in St. Lucia include Noel Venner, Leton Thomas, and Clifton Huntley.

Back in Wisconsin, we were also very fortunate to work with a team of able, loyal research assistants, including Michael Booth, Jennifer Gerner, Steve Gordon, Jane-yu Li, Lucien Lombardo, Daphne McDaniel, Henry Rempel, Geoffrey Rotwein, William Scanlon, W. Robert Schmidt, Roger Selley, and Hugo Vega. Miss Mollie Heath (now Mrs. James Bowers) was for two years not only a devoted and efficient research assistant but also performed the roles of office manager, supervisor of coding operations, and, in general, "girl Friday"; her absence during the final year of the project was genuinely felt. We want to thank all of these people, and also Professor Wilfred Malenbaum and Dr. Ben Essex, whose comments on an earlier draft of this manuscript were very helpful in our revision.

I wish also to thank my co-authors for making this joint study an example of how satisfying a truly cooperative effort can be—with everyone joining the struggle to produce a cohesive, integrated study. To Ralph Andreano I give special thanks. His contribution went far beyond the authorship of particular chapters and the careful reading of others; he shared fully with me the responsibility for organizing and shaping the work of five authors into its present form.

BURTON A. WEISBROD

Madison, Wisconsin
December 1972

Part I

THE NATURE
OF THE PROBLEM:
BACKGROUND
AND SETTING

1

DISEASE AND ECONOMIC DEVELOPMENT: THE PROBLEMS AND ISSUES

Introduction

Low income and high prevalence of disease are strongly and positively correlated, both within advanced nations and among lesser-developed parts of the world. In many areas, the incidence of a single disease such as malaria, schistosomiasis, or onchocerciasis has been thought to have profound effects on economic and social life. However, the consequences of these diseases are not well understood; it is the objective of this study to examine the nature and forms of these consequences and, to the extent possible, quantify them. We have chosen the island of St. Lucia and the parasitic disease schistosomiasis—or, as it is also known, bilharziasis—to serve as our case study.

While we should be cautious about generalizing the quantitative results of such a case study, we are confident that its usefulness goes well beyond the immediate environment in which this investigation has been conducted. Our goal is thus broader than the consideration of the effects of one group of parasitic diseases in one small part of the world. It is to develop an understanding of, as well as an analytic approach which will be of value to future work on, the interrelationship of disease and economic performance. Limitations of data, the state of knowledge concerning parasitic diseases, and our own limitations in exploring this uncharted research area have helped to make our effort fall short of the larger goal.

It remains for other researchers to continue to investigate the complicated relationships with which we have grappled, in order to determine whether an approach different from ours will push knowledge closer to this goal.

Economic Issues in Disease Control and Eradication

Knowledge of the social and economic impact of a disease is useful for a number of reasons. With health affecting the behavior of a population —for example, via its productivity and mobility—and with such behavioral characteristics affecting conditions of health—via the quality of the environment, sanitation conditions, nutrition levels, and so on— interrelations clearly exist between a country's health conditions and its economic development. If the consequences of a disease were better understood, it might be discovered, for example, that the economic and social success of a disease-control program requires a complementary set of other programs designed first to win cooperation for implementation of the control measures, and then to increase employment opportunities and either to reduce birth rates or to cope with the problems associated with accelerated population growth.

Knowledge of the spectrum of probable effects of a successful disease-control program and of the likelihood of success of alternative control measures is clearly useful to development planners, both in terms of allocation of the resources of their own country and in terms of access to foreign loans. As one report by the World Health Organization put it:

In the context of development planning an appraisal of health problems from an economic point of view is required primarily for advice on the establishment of priorities within the health budget. It can also be envisaged that a private or international organization which is requested to finance a health programme by loans may well interest itself in the narrow economic returns of such a programme, e.g. by means of cost-benefit analysis. [63]

The WHO statement refers to "narrow" economic returns—by which is meant, presumably, returns accruing in monetary form. But one of the challenges to researchers is to define benefits and costs broadly enough so as to encompass the most important advantages and disadvantages of disease-control programs—as those advantages and disadvantages are seen by the people involved—and yet narrowly enough to make feasible quantitative measurement (and even valuation) of these benefits and costs. Although the primary focus of this study is on the *economic* impact of disease, we realize that economic variables interact with a variety of social variables, and we have attempted to take these into account by making quantitative estimates of a number of nonfinancial variables that may be affected by parasitic diseases.

Even if the narrowly defined benefits expected from a disease-control program exceed costs, however, severe practical problems might exist for a government seeking to finance the health program. Tax collection systems that fail to reach large numbers of persons or which are relatively unresponsive to changes in income levels or which are easily evaded may capture for the government little of the increased income generated as a direct or indirect result of improved health. Significant governmental fiscal difficulties can result, and economically efficient investments may fail to be undertaken. International organizations may be of some value in cases such as this, but frequently even they anticipate eventual reimbursement, which may be a difficult or impossible requirement for the borrowing government. This set of problems concerning the financing of public health expenditures, however, is not examined in the present study.

The benefit-cost framework can be applied to two distinguishable problems of choice regarding the allocation of resources to improvement in health. One, which we have just been discussing, involves decision about the amount of resources to allocate toward control of any particular disease—the point being that such decisions should depend on comparisons of benefits with costs. The other involves decisions about the technique by which control will be attempted. These two choices correspond to the conventional economic questions of *what* to produce and *how* to produce it. Whatever the amount of resources to be devoted to any particular disease program there will normally remain a set of alternative methods for undertaking the program. For example, a water-borne parasitic disease such as schistosomiasis might be controlled by adding chemicals to stream water, by speeding the flow of streams, by improving sanitation practices, by informing people of the importance of boiling water, by periodic use of drugs to kill parasites inside the human body, and so on. Each control technique is likely to differ in cost and also in effectiveness (benefits), and so the choice of which technique or combination of techniques to use provides another opportunity to employ a benefit-cost framework.

Having an analytic structure—involving, in this case, benefits and costs—is one thing; utilizing the structure is another. For the social and economic impact of a disease is, generally, no simple matter to assess. For one thing, there are a number of dimensions of impacts in any particular country or region: on the size and age distribution of the region's population, on its urban-rural composition, on the attitudes of its population toward social changes, on its labor productivity, and so on.

Assessment of these impacts involves, first, specifying their probable forms, and, second, quantifying their magnitudes. Actual conditions must be compared with the (unobservable) hypothetical conditions that would prevail if the disease were absent. The general approach of this study is to attempt quantitative estimates of a number of effects of specific parasitic diseases by comparing labor productivity, school performance, and birth and death rates for persons with and without the disease, but comparable in a number of other important ways. This is to assume that were it not for disease, the "ill" persons would have the behavioral characteristics of their "healthy" counterparts.

Such an assumption is less valid the greater the prevalence and severity of the given disease. This is so because of the probable consequences of large changes in social and economic variables. If the eradication or control of an endemic disease were expected to bring about a sizable increase in the labor supply, for example, the short-run result, with the stocks of land and capital unchanged, would be a drop in the economy's capital-labor and land-labor ratios, with a resulting decrease in the marginal productivity of all labor—the "healthy" as well as the "sick." It would be erroneous to assume that if such a disease were controlled or eradicated, workers who currently have that disease would be as productive as are the workers who currently do not have the disease. With an increase in total labor supply, the marginal productivity of healthy labor would be expected to fall.

Similarly, if it were found that birth rates were lower among sick women, it would not necessarily be true that a significant decrease in the amount of illness would lead to a large permanent increase in the number of births. Pressure of population growth might bring about a reduction in birth rates among healthy persons.

These examples illustrate the most difficult problem that exists for any effort to assess the social and economic impacts of disease in less-developed countries (LDCs) as distinguished from advanced countries. In the latter, the major public health diseases have already been eliminated. Those that remain have relatively small prevalence and severity, and so the elimination of any one of them would not be likely to produce important changes in death rates, birth rates, labor supply, productivity, or social or geographic mobility. Hence, it may be reasonable to assume that in advanced countries the effects of elimination of a disease could be predicted on the basis of information about the relevant current behavior of persons not having the disease.

The point is that when a disease is endemic to an area, as is commonly the case in the lesser-developed areas of the world, its elimination or control can bring about nonmarginal changes that will ramify throughout the society and its economy—and these consequences of structural change are very difficult to deal with empirically, given the current state of knowledge. General equilibrium theory in the social sciences exists at a level of abstraction which as yet has relatively little operational value.

The problem of quantifying effects of disease control in less-developed areas is serious even if the disease is not so pervasive and severe that substantial changes in factor proportions or social relationships are expected. Even if only marginal changes were anticipated, a question would remain: are prices of inputs and outputs reasonably satisfactory indicators of factor productivities and free-market valuations? A recent WHO report appears to argue the negative: ". . . developing countries have not reached a stage of stable economic organization in which present costs and prices of inputs and outputs could be used as frames of reference" [63].

In addition, recall that market prices depend in part upon the initial distribution of income and wealth. The effective demand for public health services in a less-developed country might, for example, be different if income were more equally distributed in the economy. A question therefore arises as to whether the economist should use existing market prices in his evaluation of the effects of disease control, or whether he should use the prices that would exist—assuming they could be estimated—if there were a different income distribution such as would result from a successful disease-control program.

Another difficulty in measuring the benefits and costs of health programs concerns the physical spillover effects frequently associated with investment outlays for health purposes. For example, removing parasite-carrying snails from near the beginning of a stream provides benefits not only to the people who use the stream where they are removed but also to downstream users. Thus, in counting the total benefits of this investment, one must be sure to include any productivity increase associated with better health for the downstream users.

Similarly, certain individuals may be carrying a disease to another area and infecting the people of that region. Where a contagious disease is involved, eliminating it among one group of persons has the effect of reducing incidence of the disease among others, and so the cycle of reinfection may be broken. The total benefits from curing the first group should include the benefits of better health to the second group. Thus, the short-run effect of disease control will tend to be a lower-bound estimate of its long-run effect.

Illustrations of these technological spillover effects show why public rather than private measures are needed to handle certain health problems. The value of the increased output and other benefits may far exceed the costs of the health measures in the two illustrations cited above. However, because of the public nature of the stream and the ability of individuals to move around freely within a country, the full benefits of the health measures cannot be captured through the price system and used to help finance the socially desirable investment. Consequently, unless such "public health" measures are actually approached from a public viewpoint, the investments may never be undertaken.

Another important matter that must be borne in mind in assessing the economic benefits and costs of health measures is that behavioral responses of people in LDCs may be different from responses in more-developed areas. Suppose, for example, that it was technically possible to cure schistosomiasis by taking a particular medicine. Although there may be no problem in getting people in developed countries to take this medicine, it may be very difficult to do so in some LDCs. These people may fail to appreciate the connection between the medicine and the disease—perhaps because they do not believe in "germ theory"—or they may believe that those providing the medicine wish to hurt them rather than help them. The analyst and health planner—economist or whatever —must be aware of this type of relationship and not merely estimate the cost of producing and administering the medicine as the total cost of achieving the benefits of curing the disease.

Quantifying benefits from health programs often involves the thorny problem of valuing human life. In our empirical work we will investigate the effects of reduced illness and increased longevity on labor productivity of adults and school performance of children, but this does not imply that the only benefits from better health and extended life are those measured in output terms. At the same time, consideration of the extra-economic values of longer life and better health does not necessarily strengthen the case for devoting scarce resources to disease control nor, certainly, to control of any particular disease. Lives can be prolonged and morbidity cut in many ways: by dealing with any of the frequently numerous diseases found in less-developed areas, by improving diets, by improving housing quality, or even by increasing road safety.

Closely related to the problem of valuing life is one of the most difficult issues that must be dealt with in the public health field, especially as it relates to LDCs: the potential conflict between improved health and increased per capita output. Even if reducing the incidence of disease were to raise total output, income per capita might decrease because of population growth and the pressures of diminishing returns. Whether this effect would be offset by greater labor efficiency or other favorable by-products of improved health is one of the major factual questions to be studied. But, even if it were clear that per capita income would fall as a consequence of certain health measures, does this mean, since raising per capita income is the usually expressed goal of development-oriented government activities, that such health measures should not be introduced? A very different position is implied in the preamble of the charter of the World Health Organization which states that "the enjoyment of the highest attainable standard of health is one of the fundamental rights of every human being without distinction of race, religion, political belief, economic or social condition." If this dictum were followed literally we would undertake a massive shift of resources away from the production of other goods and services into the health field. We might all end up ignorant but at least in good health.

It seems evident from the public health activities being undertaken in less-developed countries that the per capita income goal is sometimes subsidiary to the goal of preventing disease and premature death. The feeling seems to be that if health measures lower per capita income, then this is a cost that must be accepted. Such a view, however, does not imply willingness to make unlimited sacrifices of other services and material comforts until everything that is technically possible is done to improve health standards. When Gunnar Myrdal says that people in less-developed countries are moving toward the moral imperative that "All that can reasonably be done to combat disease and prevent premature death must be done, regardless of the effect on population growth" [238, p. 1617], he leaves unanswered the key question: what is "reasonable" for a country to do in the health field? Presumably, this is a question that must be settled on a political level, given an understanding of the costs and benefits of alternative actions. It is in this area of providing information on alternatives that the social scientist has an important role to play.

Conceptual Problems: Disease and Development

The approach to be used in investigating the socio-economic impact of disease on development is based largely upon the notion of health services as a form of human investment. First made popular in the 1830s and 1840s by such writers as Edwin Chadwick and William Farr and then extended by modern writers in the human-resources field (see chapter 2), this involves distinguishing between health services as consumption goods and as investment goods. They are often investment goods because improved health conditions tend to raise labor efficiency, that is, increase the stock of human capital, and, therefore, the volume of potential output of the economy. However, many health services may be thought of as consumer goods, for they provide utility directly by reducing the discomforts of illness, quite aside from their possible effects on productive efficiency.

Economists' emphasis on the investment aspect of health services is due in part to the belief that this aspect of the benefits from health programs is not sufficiently understood from both an analytical and empirical viewpoint, and in part to the strong policy interest in raising economic growth rates. An especially important issue that this investment focus helps to clarify is whether less-developed countries are allocating funds between physical-capital projects and human-capital projects in a manner which best helps to attain their development goals.

The output increases due to improved health services can be divided into those that stem directly from individuals enjoying better health and those that flow from productive agents indirectly affected by the improved health services. The direct effects are: (1) increases in "outputs" due to the decline in absenteeism from work and school because of illness; (2) output increases associated with the rise in efficiency because of greater physical and mental ability of children and adults; and (3) output increments due to extension of working lives. Indirect effects include: (1) reductions in the goods and services required to *care* for the sick; (2) increases in output resulting from freeing of resources previously used by healthy people to *avoid* sickness [61]; (3) the output resulting from any population increase due to a rise in the birth rate, as might result from better health conditions; (4) any net output resulting from changes in attitudes and in social and political organization that might be a consequence of better health conditions.

Awareness is growing of a strong relationship between disease and economic development in the less-developed regions of the world. One form of the relationship involves the effects of developmental activities on the prevalence of such water-borne parasitic diseases as schistosomiasis, the disease to which our quantitative efforts are principally directed in this study. The connection between economic development and the prevalence of a disease may be close enough to bring despair:

. . . there is a cruel equation at work in the world: "Irrigation or malnutrition; malnutrition or schistosomiasis." In Southern Rhodesia, a $9 million irrigation project had to be abandoned before it was completed, because of the speed with which it carried [disease-transmitting] snails to previously uninfested sections of the country. The giant Aswan dam, designed to increase Egypt's arable land by a third, may unleash debilitating disease to an extent that cancels out the economic benefits of the dam. [158]

Similar results have occurred in the Middle East, particularly the Sudan and Egypt, in the Philippines, in Brazil, and perhaps even in St. Lucia, as we discuss later [154] [157]. During the past fifty years, the proportion of agricultural production originating from irrigated lands has risen markedly in all parts of the world, and perhaps increasingly so since World War II, so it is not difficult at all to believe that this has been an important contributing factor in the increase of the world-wide prevalence of schistosomiasis. The limits of irrigation use in agricultural production have probably not yet been reached, and this does not portend well for those parts of the world where the pattern of agriculture requires ditching and/or irrigation schemes and water-supply power dams.

Even if development efforts, such as expanded irrigation, do not *extend* disease, the presence of disease may well retard economic growth. The favorable productivity effects of additional capital stock, for example, may well be small if that capital is to be utilized by a disease-weakened labor force. Again, in Egypt: "Over a period of years, 22 percent of Army recruits from lower Egypt have been rejected for physical defects, whereas only 3 percent of those from upper Egypt have failed to pass the physical examinations. This wide difference is believed to be due almost entirely to the high schistosome [parasite] infection rate in lower Egypt" [159].

Not only may physical vitality be diminished by disease, but also mental achievement; mental retardation of victims of water-borne disease in Egypt is estimated to be two and one-half years by the age of eleven [132].

Such asserted effects should be regarded as hypotheses, however, not as demonstrated facts. Indeed, there has been extremely little careful research on these matters.

The Scope and Method of This Study

It will not be possible to deal directly with all the problems and issues we have discussed within the confines of a single study. Our approach is conditioned by the belief that some systematic analytical structure must be superimposed on the questions, otherwise the investigation will fall hopelessly into a collection of interrelationships which can never be disentangled and for which social scientists can add little of practical value.

Our objective in this study, therefore, is to set forth and then to implement a systematic approach for examining—quantitatively, to the extent possible—the economic and social impacts of disease. Rather than lay out an abstract methodology, however, we have chosen to concentrate on demonstrating the approach by actually applying it—to a specific disease in a specific less-developed area. Since the disease, schistosomiasis, is of large and growing importance throughout much of the tropical and near-tropical world, our findings about this disease may be of importance in their own right.

Our empirical work is concentrated on the effects of schistosomiasis, but to discover these effects involves controlling for the influence of other diseases, since in St. Lucia, as in less-developed areas generally, poverty manifests itself in the presence of many public health hazards and widespread prevalence of numerous diseases. Thus, efforts have been made to assess the impacts of several diseases caused by other parasites that are prevalent in St. Lucia—specifically, hookworm, *Ascaris, Trichuris,* and *Strongyloides.*

The fact that many people in less-developed areas are victims of more than one disease has two important, related consequences. One is that it is difficult to determine quantitatively the effects of any one disease. The other is that the control or even elimination of a single disease may or may not bring about large economic or social effects. This should be regarded, however, as a hypothesis which should be, and will be, tested.

The format for the remainder of this book is as follows: after surveying previous research on the relationships between health and economic development in chapter 2, we will present factual and institutional background information about the case-study geographic area, St. Lucia, and our case-study disease, schistosomiasis, in chapters 3 and 4. Chapter 5 and Appendices B, C, and D are devoted to quantitative assessment of the effects of schistosomiasis and other parasitic diseases. Three types of disease impacts will be investigated: demographic effects—influences on birth and death rates (Appendix B), school-performance effects on children (Appendix C), and labor-productivity effects (Appendix D). In chapters 6 and 7 we will discuss the meaning and implication of our findings in an attempt to bring our results into larger perspective. Finally there are appendices dealing with the representativeness of our data (Appendix F), with some evidence on the labor-supply function in St. Lucia (Appendix G), and with the possibility that economic development has itself served to spread schistosomiasis in St. Lucia (Appendix H).

2

THE ECONOMIC AND
CULTURAL IMPACTS
OF DISEASE:
A SURVEY
OF THE LITERATURE

Introduction

The characteristics and effects of man's diseases have long fascinated scientists. Much of the early development of modern statistical methods first used data about man's diseases. In the eighteenth century the French mathematicians, Bernoulli and La Place, both used hospital records in their research on the theory of probability [19]. Related to the early measurement attempts was the use of quantitative methods in the development of medical science itself. A happy conjunction between growing sophistication in quantitative techniques in science and technical advances in medical science occurred during the nineteenth century. It was not long thereafter that this knowledge was put to practical use to fight diseases, epidemics, and the entire mortality experience of man [19]. Improvement in crude mortality rates occurred on a wide scale in the Western industrialized nations in the nineteenth and twentieth centuries, and especially so after 1870. Improved sanitation and public hygiene were mainly responsible for this improvement [21]. But after 1870 and especially after 1900, giant strides in medical science in the advanced Western countries added years to average life expectancy at a rate unprecedented in man's history [34]. Between 1900 and 1960, for example, average life expectancy of males at birth in the United States increased from 43.7 years to 67.0 years, and this experience was equalled, and in some cases exceeded, in virtually all the industrialized nations of the West [21]. This degree of life expectancy has yet to be experienced in less-developed countries, though giant strides are being achieved in reducing mortality [21].

The Role of Disease in Economic Development Theory

Although it was clear that disease was both a cause and a consequence of low levels of social and economic development, early economists placed greater emphasis upon the latter of these two relationships. Malthus, for example, in his famous *Essay on Population* concludes after a sweeping survey of population growth throughout the world that "insufficiency of subsistence" is a principal cause of diseases, epidemics, and plagues and that these conditions in turn operate as positive checks to population increases [236, p. 514]. Classical economists also recognized, however, that disease affected the efficiency of labor. Thus, the notion that health services are a form of investment in human resources is clearly appreciated by J. S. Mill: "The labour of a physician or surgeon, when made use of by persons engaged in industry, must be regarded in the economy of society as a sacrifice incurred, to preserve from perishing by death or infirmity that portion of the productive resources of society which is fixed in the lives and bodily or mental powers of its productive members" [17].

Despite awareness of the two-way relationship between disease and development, classical economists did not stress this interaction in their development theory, nor were they especially active in urging the adoption of governmental measures to improve health conditions. Their attitude in the policy field probably was conditioned by the dependence of classical economics on the Malthusian population principle. In classical development theory, when wages are already near the subsistence level because of the Malthusian principle, a reduction in the death rate that is brought about by reducing the prevalence of a particular disease lowers wages still more and thereby merely increases the susceptibility of workers to other diseases and to malnutrition. Consequently, in prescribing public policies, classical economists emphasized the need for measures that would increase the rate of (physical) capital accumulation, since a higher accumulation rate raises wages and indirectly reduces the general incidence of diseases.

In Marxian development theory, the working and dwelling conditions of nineteenth-century England that health officials considered to be major causes of disease are themselves regarded as consequences of the economic system. According to Marx, the competitive struggle among capitalists for economic survival forces capitalists to increase their degree of exploitation of the working classes by such means as lengthening the working day, worsening working and housing conditions, and employing women and children [15]. Moreover, under a capitalistic system, public efforts to improve working and housing conditions can—on the basis of Marxian reasoning—only bring temporary relief at best. Marxists contended that the basic social relations of production between capitalists and workers must be changed to socialism before such conditions could be permanently corrected. Since Marx did not accept the Malthusian population principle, he was not concerned that the beneficial effects on the poor of establishing a class-less society would be offset by the pressure of population growth—resulting from reduced death rates—on living standards.

By the latter part of the nineteenth century, when the neoclassical tradition dominated most economic thinking, economists clearly recognized the significance of the interactions between health conditions and development. Alfred Marshall, for example, devotes a chapter of his famous *Principles of Economics* to "The Health and Strength of the Population" and points out that "health and strength, physical, mental, and moral . . . are the basis of industrial wealth; while conversely the chief importance of material wealth lies in the fact that when wisely used, it increases the health and strength, physical, mental, and moral, of the human race" [14]. However, being mainly concerned with economic problems in the comparatively rich, industrial countries in which public health conditions had improved considerably over those existing in the early part of the century, Marshall and other neoclassical economists did not make health conditions a key part of their development theory. Instead, they considered accumulation of physical capital and the acquisition of technological knowledge as the main sources of economic growth.

The views of neoclassical writers like Marshall dominated the thinking of most economists with respect to the problems of economic development until the post-World War II period. Thereafter, in response to sharply increased interest in the socio-economic problems of less-developed nations, economists began to devote more attention to the interactions between disease and development. The sharp death-rate decline in many LDCs due to the discovery and relatively low cost of new drugs and insect-controlling chemicals focused renewed attention upon the problem of population pressures that had been raised by Malthus. At the same time, studies by health officials suggested that endemic diseases cut the efficiency of labor in developing countries, and also suggested that the low living standards associated with low development levels contributed to the high prevalence of disease.

In much the manner that Edwin Chadwick had done more than a hundred years earlier, the post-World War II writers in development found it useful to think of disease in terms of a vicious circle of poverty. However, they also included such factors as low educational levels, underdeveloped natural resources, and low amounts of physical capital per worker among the causes and consequences of poverty [16]. Both economists and development planners in this period regarded the acquisition of physical capital as the crucial factor in accelerating growth rates.

Two related developments have tended to increase the significance attached to human factors in the growth process by economists and development planners in recent years. One is that statistical analyses of the sources of growth in developed countries over the last seventy-five years and the postwar experience of the developing countries have indicated the accumulation of physical capital to be much less important as a growth source than previously thought [7] [13] [59]. Human factors such as the level of education and training embodied in the labor force seem to account for much of what was formerly attributed to physical capital. The second development has been the conceptualization of these human factors into a framework that enables them to be viewed in the same manner that physical capital has traditionally been viewed. In particular, expenditures on education and health are now generally regarded as representing not only a consumption expenditure but also an investment in human resources that contributes to the economy's productive capacity. Although this notion of human capital can be traced back at least to Sir William Petty's writings in the latter part of the seventeenth century, it has not been widely used by economists in their theoretical and empirical work until very recently. This can probably be accounted for by the lack of reliable statistics that would enable investigators to compute rates of return on investment in human resources, as well as the previously mentioned view that the accumulation of *physical* capital was the key to economic development. Although most of the recent analysis of investment in human resources has been directed at education, several scholars have demonstrated how investment in health can be analyzed within the same general framework [31] [49] [61] [62].

Sociologists and social anthropologists have also made important recent contributions to our understanding of the problem and consequences of improving health conditions. In particular, they have shown that successful health programs must involve much more than simply providing medical and sanitary facilities. In order to obtain the maximum utilization of these facilities it is necessary first to understand the general culture, institutions, and beliefs of the people to whom the physical facilities are directed, and then to carry out health programs in ways that harmonize rather than clash with the prevailing cultural patterns. Otherwise there is a likelihood that those for whom the program is designed may not utilize the facilities and techniques that could bring real improvements in health [212].

As the survey of disease studies in subsequent sections will show, rigorous studies of either an economic or sociological nature have been applied almost exclusively to developed countries. Moreover, there have been no studies in which economists have combined their talents with sociologists and anthropologists, let alone with physicians, engineers, and administrators in the public health field. Yet, as Gunnar Myrdal points out, there is a pressing need for much more specific and carefully supported knowledge about facts and causal relationships with respect to health conditions in the less advanced, poorly developed countries of the world where these conditions dominate the quality of life [51] [238].

Early Studies of the Impact of Disease

In the Western nations, modern awareness of the interrelationships between health, income, and welfare started in earnest around 1830. The period 1830–1860 was rich both in quantity and in quality of studies concerned with questions of public health and clinical medicine [19]. In Europe, Great Britain, and the United States, numerous researchers investigated the problems of health and disease under a wide variety of conditions and circumstances. Many were official inquiries; others were done by individual scientists motivated by the magnitude of the health problems that confronted the industrialized nations of the West. Studies ranged from analyses of differential rates of mortality by age, sex, residence, and specific disease, to the effects of general and health conditions on economic and social class, occupation, race, imprisonment and crime, low income and poverty, intemperance, and housing and living conditions. From this point on, until World War I, studies on disease and its various potential impacts continued to be conducted. Out of this grew not only the public health and sanitation reforms commonly associated with these studies, but also considerable speculation on the role that disease and health played in national economic development. While studies continued during the interwar period, it was not until after World War II that serious and detailed research on health and disease was once again undertaken, particularly in the context of its relevance to economic growth and development.

Early studies, particularly those by the sociologist Edwin Chadwick and the medical statistician William Farr, recognized the human-capital implications of poor health and premature death [5] [10]. The economist Sir William Petty, perhaps the first to use the notion of human-capital for analytical purposes in the health area, calculated (1) the rate of return on removing the London population outside the city during epidemics of the plague; (2) the cost-benefit ratio of hospitals for illegitimate births; (3) the benefits from immigration and migration; and (4) the benefits in human lives saved, and thus the increase in national wealth, from improvements in medical care [18].

Petty's was a sophisticated and compelling argument, but so far as one is able to determine, it had little impact on other economists and on public policy. It remained for Chadwick to unite the concept of human capital with health and disease factors into an effective set of public policy recommendations. Chadwick's *Report on the Sanitary Condition of the Labouring Population of Great Britain* (1842) represented four years of careful field investigation and a much longer period of concern for the apparent social costs that the Industrial Revolution had wrought on England [5]. Chadwick's *Report* is the first systematic attempt to link disease and health factors directly to economic, social, and demographic variables. The study developed four principal points:

1. The correlation between environmental variables—insanitation, defective drainage, inadequate water supply, and overcrowded housing—and disease, high mortality rates, and low expectation of life.

2. The economic costs of ill health, which Chadwick, in a single chapter of barely twenty pages, linked directly to Petty's concept of human capital and its importance to the growth and level of national income.

3. The social costs (crime, low moral standards, etc.) of poverty and especially poor housing.

4. The lack of existing public policy and administration to deal effectively with (1)–(3).

The economic sophistication of Chadwick's *Report* is surprisingly modern, although on the whole the statistical methods used are largely descriptive: it is the conceptual framework Chadwick used that gives cogency to the massive statistical data and not vice versa. Chadwick's *Report*, and his subsequent writings and lobbying, led ultimately (in 1848) to the passage of the Public Health Act, a landmark in the history of public health movements [19] [5].

In the United States, Chadwick's energy and zeal were duplicated in the excellent studies Lemuel Shattuck conducted in Massachusetts, and especially his *Report* for 1850 [4] [47] [20]. Studies of this kind, perhaps not of comparable quality and depth, multiplied in the United States, though one in particular, for New York City, comes closest to equaling Chadwick's [6]. In Europe, especially France and Germany, there were also a number of studies of high quality at this time; Max Pettenkofer's work, with its explicit recognition of the benefit-cost framework, deserves to be mentioned [58]. Common to all these studies was the analytical concept that man had capital embodied within him and that to improve the physical conditions under which man lived was a positive public benefit. To handle this framework required use, however limited in scope and sophistication, of the concept of human capital and explicit recognition of the calculations involved in benefit-cost analysis [56] [32].

It is in this connection that the work of William Farr must be understood [10]. In a paper published in 1853, Farr calculated the money value of man, not by using the costs of rearing children or of producing a member of the labor force, but from the future income stream of workers of different ages discounted to the present. Farr was also careful to subtract consumption expenditures from his calculation, a procedure not fully appreciated until virtually the present. This surprisingly modern use of human-capital theory was regrettably ignored for the better part of half a century [33].

From approximately the latter three decades of the nineteenth century on, studies of the economic implications of health and disease became increasingly separated from various national public health reform movements in the advanced Western industrialized countries. This is not to say that such studies were not useful to these movements: rather, emphasis shifted to study of particular diseases, in particular areas, and for particular purposes, including stirring up municipal or national governmental support for public health reforms, especially in non-Western, nonindustrialized countries [135] [29]. In the first twenty-five years of the twentieth century, the United States was the principal focus for these studies. The well-known American economist Irving Fisher contributed several interesting studies, but most of the work was done by epidemiologists, parasitologists, other social scientists, and not infrequently by public health officials in local, state, and national government [33] [34] [56]. While analysis of mortality costs from premature death continued to be an important avenue of research, the focus from the beginning of the twentieth century on began to shift in various ways—toward the disability and debility effects of diseases, toward diseases of world-wide importance, and toward economic and demographic variables [130] [8] [37] [45] [123].

With one or two exceptions [28] [10], particularly Fisher's 1909 *Report* [33], the concept of human capital used to estimate disease costs continued to utilize the "cost of rearing children" approach [39] [53]. Fisher included in his estimate of disease costs the cost of premature death measured by Farr's method of capitalizing the present value of net future earnings, working time lost due to sickness, as well as the costs of medical inputs. Fisher did not, however, subtract consumption, as Farr had done.

One of the most interesting features of Fisher's work was his grappling with the measurement problems imposed by disability and debility [33]. This problem had three dimensions: (1) measuring real productivity of workers, (2) measuring the effect of working time added to total output, and (3) measuring the effect of disease control and eradication on the supply curve for labor [30] [49]. The combined measurement of mortality and debility effects of disease on labor efficiency, labor supply, and total output led ultimately to viewing disease-control and eradication programs in a context of benefits accruing through national income and adding to the national wealth stock [7] [60]. Thus, by the time of the Great Depression, and certainly by the end of World War II, application of the concept of human capital to problems of health and disease had touched on all the economic aspects that the most recent literature has suggested to be most significant [32] [49] [56]. Three distinct types of measurements emerged from this literature, and all three are useful today, though in a far more sophisticated and rigorous sense. These are:

1. The costs of rearing a child and/or of developing a productive member of the labor force. While earlier studies used this approach to justify the economic returns from better health, this measure seems now most useful when integrated with other data in assessing the burdens a high infant mortality rate imposes on an economy [109].

2. The capitalized-earnings approach, where the present net value of future work (measured through lifetime income streams), is used to calculate mortality and debility costs in terms of lost labor efficiency and decreased labor supply [28] [50] [67].

3. Measurement, by a variety of techniques, of the contribution of improved mortality, disability, and debility to the level and rate of growth of national income and product [7] [25] [26].

Modern Studies

Modern studies on the economic impact of disease have been stimulated by a number of interrelated events. First, and perhaps most important, has been the world-wide concern with the startling gap in levels of health between the Western industrialized countries and those in the less-developed world [65]. Low life expectancy, high mortality, continued persistence of epidemics and widespread infection of populations with parasitic diseases, all dramatize the glaring differences in living standards between developed and less-developed countries in a way not possible from comparisons alone of income per head [56] [20] [239] [64]. Considerable resources thus began to be invested in disease-control and eradication programs in LDCs, and some (such as malaria) on a world-wide basis [63]. It soon became clear that unforeseen demographic effects, notably accelerated rates of population growth due principally to rapid decline in crude mortality rates [21], and related economic effects (on the supply of labor, employment, unemployment, and disguised unemployment) needed to be considered in connection with proposed disease-eradication and control programs [237] [52]. It also was quickly perceived that costs and benefits could vary substantially among the technically available alternative methods for disease control or eradication [40] [65].

A second stimulus to recent research on the economic impact of disease—not related to health conditions in LDCs—was the development of public expenditure theory in industrialized nations. Conceptual and empirical work on the value of human capital created by education quickly spilled over into health variables, and these in turn were united with the growing national concern to allocate resources into programs that created a greater stock of human capital [31] [42] [61] [62] [66]. Public expenditures, given the wide range of choices of action available, required some methodological framework in which rational decision-making could take place. It was in this context that cost-benefit analysis was refined as a decision-making tool, and it was inevitable that it should also be used in the economic analysis of the value of human capital created by health care [62] [66].

A third stimulus to recent research on the economic impact of disease —related to the second—was the renewal of concern about the factors contributing to economic growth. Increased attention has been paid during the past decade to factors affecting the quality of labor inputs; again, education received the bulk of notice, but health expenditures have also been considered [7] [13].

The results of these three stimuli were a considerable amount of empirical work undertaken both in LDCs and advanced industrial countries in the past two decades on the mortality costs of specific diseases, on the benefit-cost ratios for various preventive health programs, on the labor-productivity effects of disease and health programs, and on the national income and growth consequences of improved health and reduced impact of disease [31] [42] [46] [7] [25] [26].

The quality of this work varies widely. A number of studies have asserted dramatic benefits of improved health in LDCs. Hard evidence and careful analyses are, however, scarce. Some investigators understandably wish to dramatize the potential benefits that disease-eradication programs can yield, and thereby generate support for devoting additional resources to programs of sanitation and public health. However, an absence in these studies of carefully constructed models and/or proper specification of all the costs and all the benefits renders most of them of only limited scientific use. In the specific case of measures of labor-productivity gains, for example, before and after disease eradication, there is considerable confusion of average with marginal productivity [65]. Specification of other variables such as education and diet that affect worker performance are also usually ignored, and few if any effects are assigned to social and cultural factors, a point we shall develop in the next section. Finally, account is rarely taken of the possible interrelationships among diseases in affecting worker efficiency [65].

One study of schistosomiasis in the Philippines, for example, used clinical examination of a sample population to measure absences from work attributable to the disease [138]. For four different classes (from *no absence* to *confined in bed*) an "assumed loss of working capacity" was assigned, ranging from 25 percent to 100 percent. From this the investigation then proceeded to calculate the man-days lost per annum per person infected. This sum was then valued at the "minimum wage" and added to an estimate of treatment costs (medicinal inputs and labor costs only) to arrive at the "economic loss" attributable to schistosomiasis.

One does not know what is being measured by this procedure: How was the "assumed loss of working capacity" calculated? Which, if any, of the other variables affecting the efficiency of labor were held constant? Do workers with disease have the same marginal productivity as those without it? If all the worker man-days had not been lost, would the level of total output have been different than it was with the infected workers? Why value the man-days lost at the minimum wage instead of the value of the marginal product? Are they the same? If the added output as a result of reduction in man-days lost had been large, could it have been sold at existing product and factor prices? In short, there are a number of unanswered but important questions that require answers before one can assess the economic burden of schistosomiasis in the Philippines. Yet at the same time it is true that studies such as this one for the Philippines represent a step in the evolving process of research on the economic and social effects of disease.

A significant methodological and substantive improvement over studies of the kind noted above has been accomplished in the work of Robin Barlow and Peter Newman on the economic and demographic effects of malaria eradication [25] [52]. Newman constructed a model splitting the causes of population growth into two separate but additive components:

that due to malaria eradication and that due to all other causes taken together. The model was applied to Ceylon and Guyana; Newman's results attributed about 60 percent of the acceleration in the rate of population growth in Ceylon between 1931–46 and 1947–60 to malaria eradication, and about 40 percent in Guyana. These results suggest that the economic impact of malaria eradication could be quite large, the precise magnitude depending on an incredibly complex set of interactions and interrelationships between sources of population change and sources of income and output change.

The simultaneous and general equilibrium dimensions of Newman's measurement problem were considered directly by Barlow in his related study of malaria eradication in Ceylon [25] [26]. Barlow constructed a general equilibrium model for the Ceylonese economy using Newman's population results. He then attempted to simulate income per head with and without malaria effects. In the short run, Barlow's model shows that the positive effects on output and income per head from malaria eradication are quite strong, but in the long run the negative effects—mainly population growth, resulting from eradication—which require more public resources and thus reduce government savings and the investment component, begin to outweigh the positive ones.

It should be made clear that both the Newman and Barlow studies are substantial methodological advances over previous work. But the difficulties their studies reflect indicate how complicated the interconnections are between economic and demographic effects on the one hand and health and disease variables on the other.

A recent attempt by Wilfred Malenbaum to grapple directly with the productivity of labor effects from improved health in LDCs is further illustration of the difficulties faced by researchers in this area [46]. Malenbaum applies a multiple regression model to a group of twenty-two countries and separately for Mexico, Thailand, and India. He finds an impressive relationship between various health variables (defined below) and labor productivity in all cases except Thailand and India. But one must be cautious indeed in interpreting these results. Among the health variables that are used, some—such as vaccinations against smallpox—are inputs and others—such as infant mortality—are outputs.

It is indeed difficult to distinguish between the hypotheses that low labor productivity causes poor health and that poor health causes low labor productivity. The studies by Barlow, Newman, and Malenbaum all relied on particular assumptions concerning the direction of the causal relationship between health and economic variables. A recent study by James Knowles, however, has attempted to frame a set of simultaneous equations for health and economic-demographic variables after having first developed a set of theoretical relationships postulating the causal connections between the two. The household model is estimated with Chilean data and seemingly predicts quite well the relationship between health and income per head [43].

Turning next to works applying benefit-cost analysis to health problems, a most interesting literature exists for advanced countries. Various studies have illustrated the usefulness of carefully constructed cost-benefit models to problems of public policy [31] [42] [50] [61] [66]. These studies have also suggested that the stock of human capital locked up in man's diseases, especially in the Western countries, is substantial. They have also disclosed considerable variability in rates of return on resources devoted to elimination of these diseases, although levels are uniformly high compared to alternative uses of the same resources. In this connection linear programming models may also prove to be a useful policy tool, enabling one to select a control program (or even a particular disease to eradicate) which yields the largest impact to whatever objective function is being maximized [23]. It is still too soon, however, to judge whether such work will substantially affect national health policy decisions.

In the poorer and less-developed countries of the world, benefit-cost analysis has been used on a much more limited scale than in the advanced industrialized countries [40]. The method has been applied to water supply programs [126] but has not been used extensively in the evaluation of specific disease-control or eradication programs except in the naive way already noted [63] [65]. Applications of modern medical science and strenuous emphasis on public health programs in LDCs, however, have produced marked improvements in mortality rates and average life expectancy [21] [51] [65]. But public health expenditures and disease-control programs have presented some problems, especially higher rates of population growth, that could have been foreseen had adequate models of health and economic and demographic variables been applied, as was indicated by our earlier discussion of the work by Newman [237] [21].

It is easy to be too critical, however, of these research efforts for LDCs: the magnitude of their disease problems is so great that exuberance in alleviating (however partially) the miserable plight of a population is both humane and understandable. Recognition of the complex and inter-related nature of health with economic and demographic effects has been hard in coming, but it is now realized. It is to be hoped that better co-ordination between economic and health plans will result [54] [55] [63].

Cultural Factors

Most studies of the economic impact of disease have paid little or no attention to socio-cultural forces. Anthropologists and sociologists studying both advanced Western and folk cultures have produced work, however, which strongly suggests that interpretations of findings regarding the economics of disease should be tempered by an appreciation of the influence of cultural values [195] [201] [212].[1] To attempt to eliminate diseases in folk cultures or to calculate the benefits of disease eradication without recognition of how disease and health are integrated into the culture of the society may be meaningless at best, and perhaps even self-defeating [191] [198] [168] [224].

Social and cultural conditions may also be important intervening factors at the level of implementing disease-control programs [215] [210] [131] —for advanced as well as for less-developed societies [201] [208] [211]. The persistence of folk medicine, for example, is difficult to cope with if one is attempting to implement disease-control programs premised on the values of Western scientific medical methods [213] [228] [229] [231].

To be sure, distrust of medical personnel often undermines the progress of health programs in less-developed societies. Yet the frequent failure of scientific medicine to achieve its aims is more directly an outcome of people's desire to preserve their way of life [213]. An unwillingness to accept scientific medicine usually reflects a feeling that the required accommodation would not be worth modifying customary patterns of behavior. This is not to say that disease-prevention or eradication programs are destined to fail in folk societies. Rather, success is more likely to be achieved when local customs are accounted for.

It is important to recognize also that socio-economic differences may be considered cultural differences. Low-income groups may be affected differently by, and respond differently to, diseases not only because they are more susceptible to such unhealthy conditions as inadequate diet and crowding, but because their values and beliefs may differ. Whereas early studies tended to attribute the commonly observed association between illness and low socio-economic status to the relative economic deprivation of those groups [3] [57] [44], later investigations have shown the importance of considering social-psychological and educational factors [109]. For example, individuals from low-income groups—having, on the average, lower levels of educational attainment—are more likely to be ignorant of proper health practices and innovations in medicine, and therefore, are more often unaware of the possibilities for curing diseases [220]. Or, low-income groups may distrust scientific medicine, either because of inequalities in power and rank that separate patient from physician [213], or because medical workers may provide inferior treatment to members of low social classes [195].

1. This section is largely drawn from an unpublished manuscript by Erwin H. Epstein.

Individuals who differ socio-economically are likely to vary in regard to life-style, values, and ways of viewing themselves and the world. Sociologists have found that middle-class individuals differ importantly in their views from working-class persons. In the United States, for example, the latter have been reported as emphasizing immediate gratification, compared to middle-class persons who tend to emphasize the deferment of immediate pleasure and gain for the attainment of future goals; the accumulation of material goods; the maintenance of property, education, and intellectual improvement; and ambition to "get ahead" [36]. In regard to personal hygiene and cleanliness, working-class people have been reported to be more casual about their habits [208, p. 15]. To medical workers, who are usually middle class and to whom working-class norms may be unfamiliar, working-class behavior may even seem unintelligible and irrational.

Related to differences in social class are urban-rural differences. Rural residents are thought to share some of the same characteristics as working-class persons, such as comparatively low educational aspirations [214]. It is not surprising, therefore, that rural people tend to suffer the same comparative deprivation in health care and knowledge as urban low-social-class groups. For example, rural schoolchildren in a variety of countries have been reported to be less informed about the nature and causes of diseases than urban pupils [217].

All this suggests that an understanding of the ways in which people are influenced by and respond to illness requires consideration of a variety of social and economic factors. All individuals do not react uniformly in any given set of circumstances, but neither is their behavior unpredictable. All individuals are organized into a "system" which conditions their interpersonal relationships, and knowing about that system for a given group of people can tell us much about how they relate to illness and stress, and to plans for reducing both.

Ever since research in the late 1920s it has been clear that the actual productivity of labor is influenced significantly by social factors—and not simply by the worker's physical capacity to produce, given the capital with which he works [221]. One of the most important of these studies —the "Bank Wiring Room experiment"—found that workers adhered to a social norm, enforced by their co-workers, as to the "proper" amount of production; as a result they actually produced far less than what they were physically capable of producing, despite financial incentives to work harder [197, p. 33] [206]. In a study of the life and culture of a rural Mexican community, Tzintzuntzan, it was observed that the peasants acted as though everything "good" was, like land, given by nature and available to be divided up, but was *not* capable of being increased through harder work [200]. These examples illustrate how work effort may, at the margin, be influenced by a host of social considerations in addition to the desire for money income or for greater achievement. Such cultural forces could dominate the constraining effects of disease, with the result that achievement at work and school, for example, might not be found to be affected substantially by disease infection.

Conclusion

This brief survey is meant to suggest that one should not be comfortable with either the methodology or the scope of the research results to date on the economic and social impacts of disease. Whatever its shortcomings, however, past research has demonstrated the complexity of the problems researchers face, and serves as a warning that caution and restraint is the best policy in evaluating research results or in implementing policy. What our survey of the literature suggests is the need for studies uniting the demographic, labor-supply and productivity, and disease impacts on micro and macro levels with evaluations of benefits and costs of alternative control programs for a variety of diseases and geographic areas. We believe that the empirical methodology of the present study is a move in that direction.

Before discussing schistosomiasis—the principal parasitic disease with which we are concerned—we will provide some background on the economic structure and performance and the social organization of St. Lucia.

3

ST. LUCIA: THE ECONOMIC
AND SOCIAL BACKGROUND

Historical Background

The geographic focus of this study of disease and economic development is a tropical isle, volcanic in origin, 238 square miles in area, and lying in the chain of the Lesser Antilles in the Windward Islands between Martinique to the north and St. Vincent to the south. (See Figure 3.1.) St. Lucia (pronounced *Saint Loosha*) is indeed a most visually beautiful country, with mountainous slopes, fertile alluvial valleys, and a circle of beaches of magnificent beauty. The capital of St. Lucia is Castries, a city of some forty thousand people, about 40 percent of the entire island population. In 1948 Castries was completely destroyed by fire, but it has since been rebuilt along more modern lines, with stone houses replacing the old wooden ones. Soufriere, the second-largest city, burned down in 1955 but now has been almost completely rebuilt. The only other sizable town on the island is Vieux Fort, located at the southern end of the island. Here during World War II a modern American air base was housed, but today, like most of the villages and towns outside Castries it consists largely of wooden buildings, although some modern concrete tourist facilities have been built very recently.

St. Lucia's climate is varied but generally mild. The relatively wet season extends from June to December, and the relatively dry from February to May. The mean temperature at Castries (recorded over a thirty-one-year period) varies from a low of 74.0 degrees in both Decem-

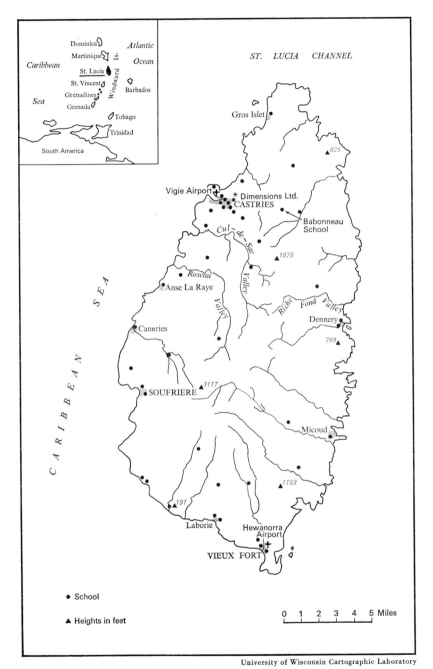

Caribbean

Sea

ST. LUCIA CHANNEL

Dominica
Martinique
St. Lucia
St. Vincent
Grenadines
Grenada
Tobago
Trinidad

Atlantic
Ocean
Barbados

South America

Gros Islet

▲825

Vigie Airport
CASTRIES
*Dimensions Ltd.

Babonneau
School

Cul-de-Sac Valley

▲1875

Roseau
Anse La Raye

Riche Fond Valley

Dennery

Canaries

▲769

Valley

SEA

CARIBBEAN

SOUFRIERE ▲3117

Micoud

▲1153

▲191

Laborie

Hewanorra
Airport

VIEUX FORT

• School

▲ Heights in feet

0   1   2   3   4   5 Miles

University of Wisconsin Cartographic Laboratory

Figure 3.1. Map of St. Lucia

29

ber and February to a high of 78.4 degrees in May. The relative humidity is high and ranges from 60 to 95 percent depending upon the time of day and the season.

English is the official language of the island but a French Creole (patois) is widely spoken, and in the villages and countryside there are still many older people who speak only this unwritten patois or who understand English only with difficulty. About 93 percent of the St. Lucians are Roman Catholic, and almost all the rest are affiliated with other denominations [181].

The island may have been settled by Europeans in 1511, when the king of Spain looked upon "Santa Lucia" as one of his possessions in the New World. But the first known attempt at settlement was made by Englishmen in 1605. This met with resistance by the Caribs, the aboriginal inhabitants of the island. A more determined effort at settlement was made in 1638; however, the Caribs again attacked the colonists, and the island was once more abandoned. The French had meanwhile developed an interest in the island, and there followed more than a century and a half of turmoil while the English and French disputed their rights to St. Lucia. Finally, the island was ceded to Britain by the Treaty of Paris in 1814 [172].

Until 1838 St. Lucia was treated as a separate administrative unit and its governor was in direct correspondence with the Colonial Office. In 1838 St. Lucia was annexed to the Government of the Windward Islands (then comprising Barbados, St. Vincent, and Tobago); despite occasional changes in the composition and seat of government of the Windward Islands, St. Lucia always remained a member. At the end of 1959, however, the post of governor of the Windward Islands was abolished, and from January 1, 1960, St. Lucia was administered as a separate unit. As of March 1, 1967, St. Lucia has had Associated Status in the Commonwealth; it is thus independent except in the areas of defense and foreign relations.

During most of the second half of the eighteenth century, the island was a small, though important, supplier of sugar to France and the American colonies. The principal mode of sugar production then, and during subsequent British rule, was slave plantation agriculture. Though legally abolished in 1834, slavery and the cultural and institutional facets of plantation agriculture continued to play an important role in the social and economic development of St. Lucia [164, p. 707], a point to which we will have occasion to refer again in later chapters.

Demographic Conditions

The exact size of the St. Lucian population is not really known [161, pp. 1–2]. A census in 1960 placed the population at about 88,000. A provisional estimate in 1965 put the population at 100,000, but the figure that most West Indians seem to accept is a population of about 110,000 as of that year. Whites of European ancestry constitute perhaps less than ½ of 1 percent of the total. Pure blacks of African origin constitute 70 percent of the population and the remainder (nearly 30 percent) consists of a small number of East Indians and a much greater number of racially mixed less dark people who are referred to as "coloured." St. Lucia, is not a white-dominated culture, but the best agricultural lands are owned by a small number of whites. The coloureds are pre-eminent in business, the professions, civil service, and only modestly so in agricultural lands. At the bottom of the social and economic pyramid are the blacks, who do most of the manual labor of the island's economy [164, pp. 710–711]. The extent to which social mobility has improved in recent years is not known but an estimate of its extent is given below in our discussion of recent changes in the island's economic structure.

The population has been growing rapidly in recent decades compared to its long-term growth rate. The long-term compound average annual rate for the period 1870 to 1960 is 1.2 percent, and experience since the last census (1960) suggests that this rate has been well exceeded in the past decade, or at least since migration to the United Kingdom was cut off by Britain in 1962. Recent population growth has thus been at 2 to 2½ percent per annum.

Net migration has not been a principal determinant of past population growth. There was one period, from 1850 to 1900, during which a positive net immigration occurred as East Indian laborers were imported to work the sugar plantations and British military troops were increased in St. Lucia to man and construct military facilities on the island. In the decade 1900–1909 withdrawal of the major portion of British troops and a large exodus of St. Lucian laborers to work on the construction of the Panama Canal resulted in negative net migration. From then until the period 1950–1962, when perhaps twelve thousand or so St. Lucians migrated permanently to the United Kingdom, the natural rate of increase determined the pace and level of population growth [167] [179].

The crude birth rate has remained fairly steady historically between 40 and 48 per 1000. In recent years the rate has been about 40 per 1000. The crude death rate, on the other hand, has fallen dramatically during the past century, and it is presently around 7–8 per 1000. This represents a drop from about 16 in 1950 and about 26 in 1915 [161, pp. 19–27] [186]. The main improvements in the crude death rates have taken place at ages 0–15. Declines in infant mortality, in particular, have accounted for most of the recent decline in crude mortality rates. As a result, the population's average age has decreased during this century.

In demographic terms, therefore, the twentieth century has witnessed some dramatic changes in St. Lucia. Like other LDCs, St. Lucia is experiencing a demographic transformation to high birth rates and rapidly declining death rates, which has resulted, especially since World War II, in what has been termed a "population explosion." Whether or not the island's resource base is sufficient to absorb this population growth without widespread unemployment and underemployment is difficult to determine. In terms of agricultural land, certain institutional problems concerning land tenure relationships and the physical geography of the island suggest that high rates of population growth may already be pressing hard against available supplies [188, p. 15].

Land pressure, in addition to the attraction of improved employment and income opportunities in urban areas, may also be an important factor contributing to the extensive rural-urban population migration that St. Lucia has experienced in recent decades. Nearly half of the island's total population now lives in the northwest corner in the Castries district. Though rural-urban migration into the Castries district has been taking place during most of the twentieth century, the trend does appear to have accelerated in recent years.

The Structure of the Economy

At first glance, the economy of St. Lucia today does not appear much different than it must have been a century ago; it is heavily dependent on a few exports as a source of income and employment, and the strongest export influence is a raw agricultural commodity, bananas [166] [175]. A hundred years ago one could have made the same statement, only substituting sugar for bananas. But there are subtle and important differences: (1) the economy has experienced some real income growth per capita in the last decade, something it was probably unable to do for any sustained period in the past, when sugar cultivation dominated the economy; (2) cultivation of bananas, because they can be grown on very small plots of ground—in one's backyard garden, for example—has permitted the development of peasant, cash agriculture to an extent never achieved with sugar; (3) the important addition of tourism income to the island's export structure has presented opportunities for income and employment growth far broader than what existed under export agriculture alone.

National income growth in St. Lucia is primarily dependent on the growth of the export sector, principally bananas and tourism. During the 1960s banana exports led an advance in the export sector which was substantial. Banana exports have leveled off in the past few years, but tourism income has expanded much faster than had been anticipated.

Estimated tourism income for 1971 was $8.5 (E.C.) million while banana exports were estimated at $5.5 (E.C.) million [163, pp. 7, 10].[1] The nominal per annum rate of growth in gross domestic product between 1964 and 1971 has averaged about 14 percent. Per capita nominal GDP was $310 (E.C.) in 1964 and was estimated at $760 (E.C.) in 1971 [163, p. 5]. Internal prices have been increasing, however, so that both real total and per capita income growth since 1964 has probably been in the per annum range of 6–8 percent. It would appear, therefore, and certainly allowing for the well-known problems connected with the construction of national income accounts in LDCs, that St. Lucia has experienced perhaps two decades of sustained income growth. Income growth in St. Lucia prior to 1948 was relatively constant and in per capita terms may even have declined between 1890 and 1948 [161, pt. 2]. That income growth appears to have been nudged off this bleak past trend makes the present period in St. Lucian history, in this one and important sense, truly unique.

THE BANANA INDUSTRY

Recent income growth in St. Lucia has been closely associated with the growth of the banana industry. For decades, sugar had been the main crop of St. Lucia. The attempt to export bananas began in 1922–1923 and was discontinued in the 1930s, but since the mid-1950s it has proved such a lucrative alternative to sugar that it now is the principal agricultural export of the island. The decline of sugar production stemmed from a variety of causes: worker strikes, inefficiency, changes in world market conditions, and entrepreneurial foresight in perceiving the market potential for bananas that was developing in the United Kingdom market [174] [38, ch. 8].

The recent transition from sugar to banana production came first on some small former sugar estates, gradually spread to peasant farmers, and ultimately to the largest of the former sugar estate lands in the Roseau, Cul-de-Sac, and Riche Fond valleys. The transformation was swift and dramatic. By 1964 no sugar was exported from St. Lucia, while bananas accounted for 85 percent of the total value of exports. A key factor appears to have been the development by Geest Industries of an organized system in St. Lucia for *marketing* bananas. The decline in sugar and the rise of bananas is shown in Tables 3.1, 3.2, and 3.3.

1. Prior to 1966, the East Caribbean (E.C.) dollar—which is the currency for all of the former British territories of the Windward and Leeward Islands—was called the British West Indian (BWI) dollar. (In spite of the official name change, the currency is still commonly referred to as "beewee" dollars.) The East Caribbean dollar is presently worth about fifty United States cents.

On the surface, banana cultivation seems to have had a dramatic effect on St. Lucia's economy and on the life of its people. Sugar cultivation in St. Lucia was historically and, up to the moment the crop was abandoned, primarily grown on large plantations. The long association of slavery and sugar plantations in St. Lucia has had an impact on the attitude of the people toward work in an employment structure of this kind. Anthropologists have suggested that the apparent antipathy toward work which many commentators have noted in St. Lucia and the West Indies in general shadows a deep resentment on the part of the agricultural population toward how and where they work and not toward work itself [170].

Table 3.1. Production of Sugar in St. Lucia, 1950–1960

Year	Number of long tons (2,240 lbs.)
1950	10,441
1952	9,203
1954	8,771
1956	10,874
1958	8,198
1960	5,448
1964	0

Source: [160].
Note: Sugar production in the entire West Indies, 1940–1960, more than doubled.

(Some implications of this attitude are discussed in chapter 6, below.) There never developed, to any great extent, a peasant class of sugar cane growers in St. Lucia. And though slavery was abolished in 1834 the widespread prevalence, historically, of the metayage system (a form of tenant farming) subsequently pushed the bulk of the agricultural population only marginally above their economic conditions under slavery [164]—at least as long as sugar culture dominated.

Banana cultivation, on the other hand, represented an opportunity for peasant farming on a scale never before experienced in St. Lucia: the crop can be grown on small plots; it does not require a long growing season as does sugar, with a ratoon (generation) of banana plants maturing on the average every nine months; the capital outlay is small; employment is non-seasonal; and it is a crop that can be cultivated on a family basis because little technical knowledge is required [178]. As a result, banana cultivation has given St. Lucia a chance to break with the slave past.

Table 3.2. St. Lucia Banana Exports, 1949–1971

Year	Volume (Thousands of stems)	Value (Thousands of E.C. dollars)
1949	.1	.1
1950	2.	4.
1951	21.	26.
1952	56.	57.
1953	143.	198.
1954	287.	490.
1955	456.	612.
1956	795.	1,579.
1957	974.	1,995.
1958	1,150.	1,946.
1959	2,514.	4,003.
1960	2,646.	3,482.
1961	3,552.	5,313.
1962	4,263.	5,860.
1963	4,508.	6,335.
1964	5,177.	8,167.
1965	6,297.	9,278.
1966	6,510.	9,141.
1967	5,870.[a]	8,453.
1968	5,727.	9,636.
1969	N.A.[b]	10,869.
1970	N.A.[b]	6,400.[c]
1971	N.A.[b]	5,500.[c]

Sources: 1949 [180]; 1950–1964 [178, p. 3]; 1965–1966 [182]; 1967–1969 [189]; 1970–1971 [163, p. 7].

[a] The 1967 export drop was due to "Hurricane Beulah," which struck St. Lucia in September 1967.

[b] Not available.

[c] A prolonged drought condition, which began in early 1970 and persisted until mid-1971, contributed to the drastic 1970–1971 export decline. An additional adverse factor during this period was the competitive demand for labor caused by the hotel construction boom. (Banana export values for 1970 and 1971 are rounded to nearest hundred thousand dollars.)

Government assistance to small farmers of bananas, and to producers of other export crops such as copra and cocoa, has been substantial, especially in recent years [163, pp. 7–9]. While the St. Lucia Banana Growers Association reports over thirteen thousand registered growers, the bulk of the banana crop continues, however, to be grown on estate-size lands, using hired labor [180]. On balance, the shift from sugar to bananas appears to have been socially productive for St. Lucia.

In the late 1960s, when the data for the present study were gathered,

Table 3.3. Export Growth of St. Lucian Banana Production

Year	Banana exports (Thousands of E.C. dollars)	Banana exports as percentage of primary agricultural exports[a]	Banana exports as percentage of total exports
1949	.1	0.0	0.0
1950	4.	0.6	0.2
1951	26.	2.4	1.1
1952	57.	4.4	2.0
1953	198.	12.9	5.9
1954	490.	24.0	13.9
1955	612.	28.6	15.8
1956	1,579.	58.8	35.3
1957	1,995.	66.1	43.6
1958	1,946.	60.6	43.8
1959	4,003.	76.3	63.2
1960	3,482.	76.6	64.5
1961	5,313.	77.8	68.7
1962	5,860.	82.3	76.7
1963	6,335.	82.1	79.6
1964	8,167.	84.6	83.1
1965	9,278.	86.4	83.1
1966	9,141.	80.7	75.5

Sources: Table 3.2 and [182].

[a] Domestic exports minus sugar.

St. Lucia was in the midst of a banana "boom." It was clear then, and has now become a fact, that continued growth of banana exports could not be sustained at that level. Two major constraints were the limits of banana consumption in the United Kingdom market and the then potential entry of Britain into the European Common Market. As already noted, banana exports, estimated for 1971 at $5.5 (E.C.) million, were about half the value of exports of 1969. In part this decline is due to drought conditions and to a slowing of the market growth for bananas in the United Kingdom. In addition, a booming construction industry, oriented toward tourism, has pulled many small banana growers out of banana production and into employment in construction [163, p. 7].

The entry of the United Kingdom into the European Common Market is likely to have positive and negative effects for St. Lucian agriculture, especially bananas. It is presently expected that when Commonwealth preferences disappear St. Lucia will become an Associated Overseas territory under Part 4 of the Treaty of Rome. With regard to bananas, St. Lucia will then have to compete with the French Caribbean Departments (Guadaloupe and Martinique) and the African Associated States. At least one careful student believes St. Lucian bananas will be able to withstand these competitive threats and perhaps even displace the presently large volume of banana exports from Latin America to the European Economic Community (E.E.C.); these latter producers now face the E.E.C.'s 20 percent common external tariff as does St. Lucia, but with the entry of the United Kingdom the St. Lucia tariff position will improve whereas the Latin American positions will not [177].

On balance, the St. Lucian economy in 1972 seems less dependent for its income growth solely on the performance of the banana industry. Tourism is booming and light manufacturing, while still in its infancy, has also been growing in recent years. Compared to the economy at the height of the banana boom (1960s), the St. Lucian economy in 1972 is somewhat more diversified and better insulated from the shock of a sudden fall in banana export income [163, p. 5]. Whatever the future may hold for the St. Lucian economy, we can conclude that the recent past, especially the last decade, has been unique in St. Lucian history. For the first time, income growth of a sizable magnitude has occurred, and the level of living for the average St. Lucian has vastly improved.

St. Lucian Culture and Customs

A number of social customs and cultural traits must be discussed as part of the essential background to this study. Knowledge of institutional forms, as we shall note in later chapters, may well be important in interpreting empirical findings. Social customs, for example, often are extremely important influences on the responses to and hence the success of disease-control programs.

Culture and customs are of concern at this point for three reasons: (1) they indicate some of the problems that were encountered in the data-gathering process which underlies the empirical work; (2) they present a somewhat broader framework than is possible from economic analysis alone for interpreting the impact of disease; and (3) they are possibly important for implementing public policy with respect to schistosomiasis control and eradication.

NAMING CUSTOMS

For anyone doing survey research in St. Lucia, where the cross-referencing and checking of family names is involved, the naming customs of the country present a rather imposing barrier [165]. Several anthropologists have studied this process, and there now is some limited agreement on how the custom works. When a St. Lucian child is born, his parents choose one godparent of each sex if he is to be baptized a Catholic, or two godparents of his own sex and one of the opposite sex if he is to be Anglican. Each godparent then chooses a name for the child, and Catholic parents normally add a third name of their own choosing. Every St. Lucian child thus has three "first names" as well as his "last name" or "title," as it is called on the island [165]. As adults the practice of frequent name changes, often related to the set of names in childhood but sometimes not, continues. Serious technical problems in legal matters have been the result, to say nothing of the problems encountered by social science researchers attempting to link data to the correctly named person [165].

THE LANGUAGE BARRIER

For more than a century English has been the language of St. Lucia's government and courts [169] [170]. Yet except for Castries—the one place on the island where English is perhaps heard more often than patois—it is possible to walk for hours in the streets, wandering in and out of homes and shops, without hearing a word of English spoken; needless to add, this is all the more certainly true of the countryside. English—being the language of government but not the most widely spoken idiom—has tended, therefore, to become associated with a privileged class of people, with those who, by virtue of education, occupation, and manner of living, stand in contrast to the peasant fishermen and laborers who form the bulk of St. Lucia's population. It has become the language of those whose familiarity with scientific advances or industrial technology now sets them apart; of those who have learned more sophisticated (and expensive) standards and tastes; of those who have traveled, incorporated foreign values, come to feel that their lives are tied up with those of people in distant places. Most important, English is pre-eminently the language of white men, those who associate regularly with white men, and those who serve the interests of unseen white men: the plantation managers, census takers, bank tellers, and sellers of expensive clothing and mechanical wares. It is not that English is despised; most St. Lucians are influenced by strong socio-economic incentives to learn it. But people who speak only English—including many physicians and health workers —are likely to be accorded little trust [169] [170].

RELIGION

Patois is one major legacy of the French occupation of St. Lucia in the eighteenth century; the second is Roman Catholicism. Indeed the religious history of the island during the past two centuries has been one of persistent low-keyed conflict between two religious orientations representing two contrasting ways of life. On the one hand have been the Protestants—tending to be wealthier, more sophisticated, English-speaking, guided by English clergymen, and oriented toward British culture;

on the other hand, Catholics—distributed more uniformly throughout the population but concentrated at the lower end of the status scale, many poorly educated and semi-literate, patois-speaking, provincially oriented, and under the guidance of basically conservative French priests.

The political and economic influence of Protestants in St. Lucia has long been disproportionate to their numbers. Although controlling only some 10 percent of the island's schools, Protestants have been influential in the education of many of the island's leading government and commercial figures, and a number of prominent political leaders (including the current governor and the premier) are Protestants. At the other end of the social scale, laborers and fishermen are Catholic almost without exception. Aside from whatever effects their religion may possibly have exercised on their personalities and attitudes, it is certain that this is another social-cultural marker of which St. Lucian people are very much aware.

SPIRITUAL BELIEFS IN ST. LUCIA

The average St. Lucian's ideas about illness appear to be a blend of folk and scientific medical concepts. Most people, especially in the older generations, approach illness with a limited range of "diagnostic" terms. Leonard Glick, an anthropologist who has made observations in St. Lucia, reports that one very often hears about *fwedi* ("coldness" or "chill") and *ápwudó* ("imprudency"), the former being ambiguously associated with a variety of organic symptoms, while the latter may refer to anything from dietary to behavioral indiscretions, and occasionally may be a more or less veiled reference to sorcery as an explanation for serious or unusual illness. But this is not to say that there is no understanding of the organic nature of illnesses; many people do seem to be aware of such common diseases as schistosomiasis, typhoid, and tuberculosis [192] [169] [170].

The existence of a variety of evil beings and powers capable of causing illness is commonly believed. The term *obeah* refers to what human beings can do to one another through sorcery and other forms of "black magic." Indeed, official cognizance of *obeah* has been taken by the government. The *Criminal Code of St. Lucia, 1957* states:

A person practicing obeah means any person who, to effect any fraudulent or unlawful purpose, or for gain, or for the purpose of frightening any person, uses or pretends to use any occult means, mesmeric or otherwise, or pretends to possess any supernatural power or knowledge. . . .

In any prosecution for an offense under this section, it is not necessary that any witness should depose directly to any precise consideration or to the fact of the offense having been committed with his participation or his own personal or certain knowledge. . . . But so soon as it appears to the Court that the circumstances in evidence sufficiently establish the offense complained of, the Court shall put the defendant on his defense and in default of such evidence being rebutted shall convict the defendant accordingly. [169, p. M-4]

The spiritual beliefs of most St. Lucians directly influence their relationships with physicians and health workers. Most people will consult a physician for prolonged illnesses, especially if a child is sick, but if the illness is sufficiently mysterious or unusual in character to suggest an "unnatural" cause, the sufferer or his family may also seek the advice of a *gadé*, a folk curer. If people are convinced that a sorcerer is behind an illness, a *gadé* may be relied upon exclusively for aid. Curiously, physicians often unwittingly foster this reliance on their competitors, the *gadés*. Not having an appreciation for folk beliefs—and being *béché* (a rather derogatory term for white men) and non-patois-speaking—most physicians have neither the time, training, nor inclination to give satisfactory attention to many St. Lucians' ills.

In contrast to the physician, the *gadé* is capable of drawing upon the values and beliefs of his patients. With the overwhelming majority of the St. Lucian population being Roman Catholic, while many physicians are British and not Roman Catholic, the *gadés* are in a position to utilize their knowledge of that religion and of ancestral folklore to good advantage.

Folk medicine cannot be dismissed as simply another obstacle to be overcome in controlling disease. It represents an integral part of St. Lucian culture and as such must be considered as having potential redeeming value, inasmuch as the health of a people concerns not just their physical welfare, but also their social and psychological well-being. To be sure, were we to use scientific criteria to evaluate the worth of a given folk practice to accomplish its avowed health ends, it would most likely fail the test. The popular plant *simé kotwa* (in patois) is frequently prescribed for (among other things) worms. To show only that that remedy is ineffective is to ignore the fact that its prescription may have an important latent function, such as maintaining a system of social control essential to the society's stability. The individual may take the remedy not because it destroys the parasites directly, but because it may help to counteract the reason believed responsible for the illness, perhaps an indiscretion committed against another person or even malevolent thoughts about him.

It is therefore clear that to assess the total physical, social, and emotional effects of schistosomiasis and its control requires the recognition of a constellation of cultural factors. Even from the traditional standpoint of enhancing physical well-being, it may be calamitous to overlook the importance of culture [165] [169] [170].

Health Conditions in St. Lucia

It may be appropriate to end this chapter and this section of the book with a brief discussion of the overall disease situation in St. Lucia. More detailed information about parasitic diseases will be given in chapter 4. What we will do now is take a broad look at health conditions in St. Lucia.

Commentators from as early as the eighteenth century have written that St. Lucia was an "unhealthy" island. The climate and health conditions have frequently been termed "insalubrious." An early medical guide to the area reports a range of disease and health conditions in St. Lucia which to one degree or another would persist in the island for a century or more: typhoid fever, yellow fever, various intermittent fevers, tetanus, various respiratory infections, dysentery and other diseases of the digestive system, hepatitis, yaws, and elephantiasis [173]. If one were to add to this early list malaria, cholera, hookworm, and other parasitic diseases including schistosomiasis, one would have a fairly accurate list of diseases that historically have affected the mortality and morbidity experience of St. Lucia. Throughout most of the nineteenth and intermittently during the twentieth century, many of these diseases appeared in St. Lucia in epidemic proportions. The great epidemiologist, August Hirsch, considered St. Lucia an endemic area for malaria, yellow fever, and typhoid fever. He reported in 1883 that consumption (tuberculosis) caused more deaths than any other disease save dysentery [233]. Whether or not St. Lucia was above or below the average level of disease in the Caribbean is difficult to say. The impression one gets is that disease was one of the most important factors affecting the character and quality of life in nineteenth-century St. Lucia [171].

Only in the most recent decades of the twentieth century have general health conditions improved in St. Lucia. Prior to the end of World War II, the nineteenth-century disease patterns continued to persist. It was, for example, the most malarious island of all the British Windward and Leeward Islands as measured by average morbidity and mortality rates [93]. Malaria was not successfully eradicated in St. Lucia until the end of the 1950s, after an extensive campaign directed by the World Health Organization. While this was certainly the most notable health advance on the island within the past two decades, other improvements in health have also occurred. At the present, St. Lucia is relatively free of yellow fever, yaws, elephantiasis, cholera, typhoid, and certain forms of dysentery, all of which had been important diseases.

Diseases of childbirth and early infancy are still important causes of mortality in St. Lucia, and though infant mortality rates have declined markedly in the past decade, these still represent major health problems [161, pt. 2].

Crude death rates have declined in the 1960s to quite respectable levels (7–8 deaths per 1,000), despite the widespread existence today of allegedly debilitating parasitic diseases. Nutrition levels have probably risen in recent years because of the growth of cash income, but they are still low by standards of good health practice. A 1961 survey revealed considerable protein deficiencies, a condition that appears to have been characteristic of St. Lucia's past nutritional status as well [98].

The extent to which St. Lucia's economic performance in the past has been affected by its experience with disease and health is not easily determined. Certainly, the high mortality and infant-mortality rates that prevailed in the early part of this century were high human costs for this society to absorb. But the potential benefits to St. Lucian national income that might have resulted from lower mortality rates must remain largely problematical: the sugar crop got harvested every year, the cocoa was made, the logwood harvested, and life, in general, changed very little. Other reports, particularly covering the period 1887–1929, show that even as mortality rates were improving, a variety of parasitic diseases, including malaria, and yellow fever were taking their toll of St. Lucians, and, one might suppose, limiting the energy and vitality of laborers. Still, what high morbidity levels must have cost the St. Lucian economy in unused and underutilized resources is largely unknown.

A number of writers on economic development have suggested that one of the principal development barriers faced as a result of early mortality is the large fraction of resources devoted to child-rearing. These resources, it has been argued, are "wasted," when, because of poor health and disease conditions, a large fraction of the children die before reaching an age at which they can make productive contributions to their society as workers. High death rates in the age group 0–15, therefore, are considered one of the costs shifted onto the entire economy because of premature death.

We have made a calculation of this child-mortality cost for St. Lucia for the years 1901, 1910, and 1960. These calculations show that nearly 6 percent of St. Lucian national income in 1901 and 1910 was consumed by children who died before reaching the age of sixteen. By 1960 the comparable percentage of national income was 1.5, reflecting the marked improvement in mortality rates for the 0–15 age group. Comparable estimates for other countries of the cost of children's mortality suggests that the St. Lucian experience in the early part of the century was unusually high. W. Lee Hansen has calculated costs as a percentage of national income by the same method and assumptions used here, for

India, the United States, and the United Kingdom in 1931 and 1951. His results were as follows: 1931: India, 2.81 percent; United States, 0.32 percent; United Kingdom, 0.26 percent; 1951: India, 2.83 percent; United States, 0.09 percent; United Kingdom, 0.07 percent [36]. These calculations show that St. Lucia has experienced high relative costs because of premature death for the population group under fifteen years of age and continues to do so in 1960. To the extent that the children that died before entering employment would have been as productive workers as those already in the work force, their premature death consumed resources that could have been used elsewhere.

Conclusion

The preceding pages hardly exhaust the rich cultural and social heritage of St. Lucia. Its historical development has been an interesting and varied one. St. Lucia is now of interest because of the presence of schistosomiasis infection and the belief that this parasitic disease may have negative effects on the productivity of workers, on schoolchildren, and on demographic trends. We turn next to a description of how schistosomiasis is transmitted and how it is believed to affect the human body. This information will serve as a basis for our hypotheses, developed later, regarding the effects of the disease on social and economic behavior.

4

SCHISTOSOMIASIS:
ITS NATURE AND EXTENT

Schistosomiasis: The Nature of the Disease

S chistosomiasis is a complex disease that is caused by parasitic blood flukes, or schistosomes.[1] The life cycle of the schistosome is one of nature's ironic and complicated accomplishments, as we will describe below. The genus *Schistosoma* has a number of species, each of which is attracted to a specific intermediate snail host and which, in turn, produces somewhat different kinds of infection in the main host, principally man but in some circumstances also animals. The three major species that affect humans are: *Schistosoma haematobium*, *S. mansoni*, and *S. japonicum*. Though the effects on man are more complicated than we can appropriately discuss here, *S. haematobium* is principally drawn to the urinary bladder, *S. japonicum* to the large intestines, and *S. mansoni* to the small intestine.

The infective stage of the schistosome parasite, in all three species, involves free swimming larval forms called cercariae (about .5 millimeter in size), which may exist in fresh water ponds and streams where man

1. This discussion is based on a variety of sources, all given in the bibliography section on schistosomiasis. For the layman [71] [77] are especially helpful. Much more technical detail on the disease in general can be found in [74]. We have tried to keep our discussion at a nontechnical level.

(or animal) comes in contact with them. The cercariae enter man primarily through penetration of the unbroken skin or, possibly, from ingestion of infested water. The cercariae, now called schistosomulae, travel via the lymphatic system through the heart to the lungs and, subsequently, gain access to the liver, where they mate and mature. Depending on sex and species of the adult schistosomes, they will range from about 6 to 25 millimeters (1 inch) in length.

The mated worms usually migrate from the liver—the destination varying according to species—prior to egg laying. About six weeks after the original cercarial infection (actually between four and eight weeks), eggs, thousands of them, are produced by the now mature worm. If the eggs accumulate in the liver in sufficient numbers, they damage the cells

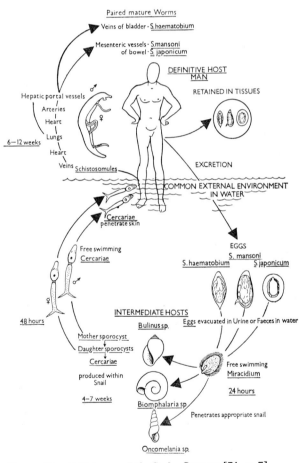

Figure 4.1.   *Schistosoma* Life Cycle. Source: [74, p. 7].

and gradually may produce internal poisoning. If the eggs infiltrate the intestinal wall, they produce hemorrhages and the absorption of food is impeded, with the consequent result, in severe cases, being diarrhea, bloody discharge, or abdominal pain. If the eggs penetrate the urinary tract, lesions of the bladder occur. In all these varieties of infection, the medical belief is that the host's body is weakened and that the accompanying fever, headache, and loss of weight in serious cases probably decrease resistance to other infection [71].

The next phase of the cycle begins when the infected host excretes the eggs. If the excreted eggs reach water they hatch a swimming embryo, called a miracidium, which in turn seeks the right species of snail and penetrates it. The now-infected snail produces sporocysts which in turn produce cercariae—completing the life cycle of the parasite.

Tremendous multiplication occurs during the schistosome life cycle. Each worm pair, in a human host, may produce several hundred eggs per day; and heavily infected persons have been known to pass tens of thousands of eggs per day. In addition, given the infection of the suitable snail species, a single schistosome egg may ultimately be responsible for roughly 1,200 cercariae. The reproductive rate of snails is also extremely high, and because of this it has been found that high prevalence rates in humans can be maintained even if as few as 1 percent of the snail population is infected [71]. (See figure 4.1.)

The "Unconquered Plague"

Schistosomiasis has been called "The Unconquered Plague." For a century, at least, the disease has resisted many of man's attempts to eradicate it.

The disease is an old one, dating, many authorities believe, from perhaps 1550 B.C. or earlier. Textual references found in the *Papyrus Eber*, first discovered near Lubar in Egypt about 1870, clearly resemble modern diagnoses of schistosomiasis. Napoleon's army in the Egyptian campaign is reputed to have contracted the disease, and for nearly two centuries since, schistosomiasis has continued to be one of man's principal parasitic diseases.

As one authority on parasites has pointed out: "A parasite's existence is usually an elaborate compromise between extracting sufficient nourishment to maintain and propagate itself and not impairing too much the vitality or reducing the number of its host, which is providing it with a home and a free ride" [71]. Schistosomiasis, to a remarkable extent, fits this characterization. Though the parasite causing the disease is an animal of a low level of genetic development, its intricate and highly specialized reproductive cycle has enabled it to survive for perhaps forty centuries or more, living off both its intermediary host (snails) and final hosts (man) without eradicating either. Though the parasite may exact a high price by debilitating or even, in extreme cases, by killing its intermediate or main host—a matter about which our empirical analyses will provide some evidence—its record for longevity and persistence is evidence of nature's impersonal and impartial ways.

Although there is much remaining to be learned concerning the conditions under which a person will develop serious clinical symptoms as a result of schistosomal infection, it seems clear that the severity of pathological effects is dependent upon both the frequency and duration of infection. Thus, standing in infested water *daily*, while bathing or washing clothes, can lead to vast levels of egg deposition in the human body over a period of years. Clinical symptoms also vary according to the particular schistosome species and according to the strain of species. Nutritional status is another factor that is likely to determine whether schistosomal infection leads to serious clinical symptoms; there is a greater probability of severe symptoms among persons with poor diets. Finally there is the weakly understood factor of host resistance; whether as a result of inherent differences in resistance or due to immunological effects of prior exposure, some groups of persons appear to tolerate the infection much better than others. For all of these reasons, the range of clinical symptoms for persons infected with schistosomiasis is broad indeed: from infections having no apparent symptoms at all, to development of abnormal livers and spleens, headache, fever, and abdominal and intestinal distress, and, ultimately, to damaged internal tissues that may have extreme effects on the person's ability to function normally.

Little is known, really, about how schistosomiasis has spread through time and whether or not the severity of infection is greater today than in previous times. Many authorities suspect that its world-wide prevalence has increased dramatically since the end of World War II. Whether or not levels of infection are accelerating, it does appear that the disease is more widespread at this point in time than a century or perhaps even fifty years ago. Two plausible explanations can be offered to permit this conclusion: large-scale migration from infected to noninfected areas has occurred, and construction of dams and greater irrigation in agriculture have probably enlarged the areas and numbers of people potentially reached by infested water.

Though some scientific knowledge of the disease's parasitological properties has existed for many years, it is only in the past two decades that the scope of scientific research has begun to reach the proportions suggested by the world-wide prevalence of the disease. Between 1949 and

1958, for example, nearly 2800 technical papers were written on the disease, and, since that time, perhaps an even greater number of scientific comments about the disease have appeared [71]. A wide variety of control experiments have been tried, some formerly endemic areas have shown improvements in prevalence rates, progress in treating infected humans has increased, but still, in 1972, man's struggle with the snail and the worm it carries continues. Much basic research remains before man can win.

World Distribution of Schistosomiasis Infection

The number of people infected with schistosomiasis is not easily calculated. During the past twenty-five years, estimates of the number infected have ranged from 100 million to 200 million persons. One careful study, however, has attempted to pool and evaluate evidence on prevalence rates from all known schistosomiasis areas. These data, shown in Table 4.1, are compiled from surveys undertaken in the period 1955–1964. These estimates, which the compiler believes to "lean too far toward the conservative side," show schistosomiasis to be endemic in seventy-two countries or

Table 4.1. World Distribution of Schistosomiasis: Population Exposed, Population Infected

Region[a]	Number of countries or islands	Total population of region	Population exposed	Population infected
Africa[b]	43	301,770,000	187,568,280	74,383,310
Mascarene Islands[c]	2	7,161,000	5,471,000	677,000
Southwest Asia[d]	9	84,386,000	9,977,300	3,232,520
The Orient[e] (except E. Asia)	6	857,856,000	101,910,000	33,309,000
The Americas[f]	11	97,033,494	49,436,000	6,302,200
Total	71	1,348,206,494	354,362,580	117,904,030

Source: [106, p. 307].

   [a] India has been omitted from this compilation because only one small focus of the disease is known to exist in that country.

   [b] *Africa* includes North (5 countries), West (19), Central (8), East (6), and South (5).

   [c] *Mascarene Islands* include Malagasy Republic and Mauritius.

   [d] *Southwest Asia* includes Aden, Saudi Arabia, Yemen, Iraq, Iran, Syria, Turkey, Lebanon, Israel.

   [e] *Orient* includes Mainland China, Japan, Philippines, Celebes, Thailand, Laos.

   [f] *The Americas* include Brazil, Surinam, Venezuela, Puerto Rico and Vieques, Dominican Republic, St. Maarten, Antigua, Guadeloupe, Martinique, St. Lucia.

islands with a total population of about 1.34 billion, of which 354 million are exposed to infection and 117.9 million are infected [106]. These data are, perhaps, the most concrete accounting one could make of the world-wide scope of infection from human schistosomiasis. The geographic distribution of schistosomiasis throughout the world is shown in Figure 4.2.

Though some countries with high infection rates of schistosomiasis have higher income per head than others, average per capita gross domestic product (GDP) in 1964 for thirty-four countries (the major areas of infection) officially declared schistosomiasis-infected was $200, an amount about equal to the world mean. The median rate of population

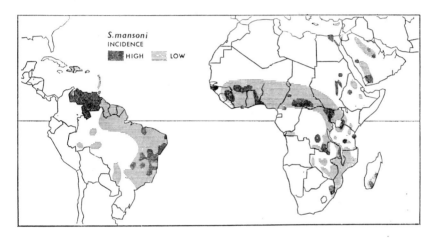

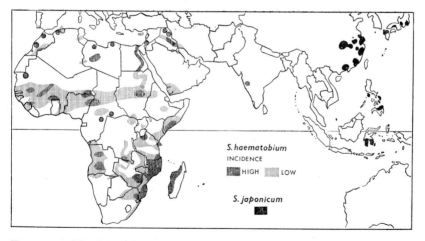

Figure 4.2. World Distribution of Schistosomiasis, 1959. Source: [76].

growth, 1958–1966, for the thirty-four countries was 2.6 percent per annum. Most of these countries also had low levels of caloric intake per day, high infant-mortality rates, and low life expectancy. Virtually all the schistosomiasis-infected countries are heavily dependent on export agriculture, and a great many of them depend on a single agricultural crop. Most of the countries exceed the world mean of 59 percent of active population in agriculture. In short, the schistosomiasis-infected countries are characterized by a high degree of dependence on agriculture, poor health, and low levels of income.

Prevalence rates and infection intensities certainly vary widely from country to country and even within regions and areas of individual countries. One study in the delta area of Egypt, noted by W. H. Wright, found ". . . significant differences in rates of infection of *S. haematobium* between sections within a division, between adjacent villages, and even between different parts of one village" [106, p. 302]. Within countries schistosomiasis seems to be of highest prevalence in rural areas where, as compared to urban places, sanitary standards are lower and access to potentially infested water sources is greater. The natural sources of water infection—lakes, rivers, ponds, etc.—tend to be greater in rural areas than in urban areas, as are man-made sources of water, principally irrigation ditches. Many studies have shown that areas under perennial irrigation are sources of endemic infection in more cases than not in LDCs [147]. The point is, therefore, that one must be cautious in making generalizations about world-wide or even country-wide prevalence levels and infection rates on the basis of a few nonrandom observations.

Transmission and Control

Water is the principal element complicating control and eradication of schistosomiasis. If man did not walk in infested water, if children did not play in it, if women did not wash clothes in it, if no one drank it, the disease would not persist in man. Similarly, if human waste was disposed of properly rather than being washed by rains into streams, ponds, drainage ditches, and water wells, or placed there directly, then the disease would also probably not persist in man, although there is, in some areas, the possibility that animal hosts could maintain the transmission cycle.

To control or eradicate the disease thus becomes intimately bound to the life-style of man and the life cycle of the schistosome parasite. Total *eradication* requires a break at some point in the transmission cycle; either the snails must be eliminated or human contact with infested water halted. Total eradication, thus, is a most difficult and costly procedure. The most desired approach, and that which has been followed in many parts of the world, is to seek *control*, to bring prevalence rates and infection down to nonappreciable levels. A break in the transmission cycle has been attempted by some combination, if not all, of the following methods: (1) by keeping the schistosome eggs excreted by humans from entering water which people use in their daily lives; (2) by eliminating the snails in which the embryos develop to larval stages; (3) by keeping the potential human victims away from infested waters; and (4) by mass chemotherapy.

Scientific and engineering research on these possibilities has been underway for many years and in many parts of the world. With respect to approach (2), a great deal of experimentation has been done. The application of molluscicides (chemicals to kill the snails) is the most prevalent method used at present, with Bayluscide and Frescon the two most popular compounds currently used in snail-eradication programs. While each of these has proven lethal to the types of snails involved in the transmission of schistosomiasis, as well as to snail eggs and larvae, they also have certain, though not fatal for control purposes, drawbacks [74, p. 185].

On a long-term basis, improved water resource planning can also contribute to the reduction of carrier snails. Such techniques as ditching to prevent stagnant water pools and reditching to speed water flows in irrigation canals are being tried, but they are costly to implement and must be maintained continually to be effective.

In recent years a great deal of medical research has occurred with respect to approach (4). Until recently, potassium tartrate antimony (and other related antimony derivatives) was the predominant "cure" for schistosomiasis. Treatment involves a series of shots given at least once per week over a period of four to seven weeks. However, the unpleasant side effects (severe nausea and vomiting) discourage large numbers of people from completing the treatment. The possibility of achieving more satisfactory results from mass treatment of the population has been enhanced, more recently, by the discovery of the drug Hycanthone. According to Peter Jordan and Gerald Webbe [74, p. 124], the drug has produced cure rates of 80 to 83 percent in certain trials. Further tests are being conducted. Regardless of the drug used, however, there are limitations to the successful application of mass drug therapy. It is difficult (and impossible in some areas) to locate and treat the entire population in an infested area.

Most authorities agree that approaches (1) and (3) offer the most promising control possibilities, and considerable experimentation is underway. Man is rational, one might argue, and if something is shown to be bad for him surely he would want to alter his behavior to avoid it.

Regrettably, it does not seem to be so simple. Keeping schistosome eggs away from water where they can hatch or keeping people away from infested water sounds uncomplicated enough. But to do so requires a level of private (and public) sanitation and health consciousness that is usually absent (or at best difficult to achieve) in the less-developed parts of the world where schistosomiasis is most prevalent. Fundamentally, it requires a population to alter its life pattern. Just as it is not easy for industrialized man to eliminate addiction to tobacco or alcohol, populations in the schistosomiasis-infected countries find it difficult to alter their customs and habits as to where they drink water, wash clothes, permit their children to play, and perform their bodily functions. So while it is true that control options (1) and (3) may offer the most promise, one can only mean that in a "second-best" sense: for these options clearly will involve tampering with the values, mores, and life-styles of people, and such programs are always difficult to introduce, whether it be in a less-developed or in a developed country.

Nonetheless, a certain amount of success in controlling schistosomiasis —principally using one or more of the options for interrupting transmission noted above—has been achieved in some parts of the world, and in others impressive control programs are now underway. Japan and Puerto Rico have had notable success in control efforts. In Venezuela, Iran, the Sudan, and the People's Republic of China large-scale control programs are being introduced. Partial control programs are also underway in Brazil, Egypt, and the Philippines, and pilot programs have been launched in Ghana, Tanzania, and Ethiopia [152]. One of the most interesting cases of large-scale control is what has apparently occurred in the People's Republic of China. Here, by employing all four possibilities for interrupting the transmission cycle, a major attempt is underway to control schistosomiasis [94].

Schistosomiasis in St. Lucia

Schistosomiasis in St. Lucia is of the *Schistosoma mansoni* species. Just when and how the disease came to the island is not fully understood. As was noted in chapter 3, St. Lucia has a long history of parasitic diseases, although medical and hospital reports in the late nineteenth and early twentieth centuries, while reporting diseases well known now, do not mention schistosomiasis. That this is so is certainly understandable: the disease does not appear to have a high mortality rate attributable directly to it; and, historically, so many other diseases were important to St. Lucian mortality experience that one could not expect St. Lucian physicians, however well trained they may have been, to have provided complete diagnostic information on all diseases.

In 1924, at any rate, definite evidence of infection was obtained when a European male in St. Lucia was diagnosed as having *S. mansoni*. Subsequently, infected snails were found at the town of Soufriere. In 1930 a survey of schoolchildren indicated that 10 percent of them were excreting *S. mansoni* eggs.

As far as one can tell, no further reports of deaths or of probable infection appeared until 1948, when a Dr. P. A. Clearkin, reporting on suspected infection sources in Soufriere, commented: "The infections seen were very light and therefore the disease is not a serious problem" [184]. And later in the same report: "A number of snails which might serve as an intermediate host did not appear to be the species which are known to act as such. And thus an aged fallacy dies a most timely death" [184].

The following year, however, a less cautious attitude prevailed. In the Soufriere area a Mr. Long carried out a series of stool examinations on a random sample of the population. His findings showed that 46.45 percent of the stools examined contained *S. mansoni* eggs. And as Long reported: "A fair percentage of the *Schistosoma* appear to be asymptomatic or, at any rate, sub-clinical but there is clearly the need for a good Public Health Programme to eradicate this disease in Soufriere" [185]. Thus it was already noted in the late 1940s that many persons who were infected with schistosomiasis had no apparent symptoms. The possibility that such a situation continues to exist in the late 1960s—a matter to which we turn in chapter 5—cannot, therefore, be dismissed.

During the 1950s a steady increase in prevalence of *S. mansoni* eggs in routine stool examinations was noted, especially in the Castries (the capital city) and Soufriere districts. A survey carried out in 1961 showed infection rates as high as 68 percent among schoolchildren in some areas, and the continued stool examinations in hospitals and health centers revealed prevalence rates of some significance for virtually all parts of the island. Though all the evidence is not yet complete, it does seem that due either to better reporting, diagnosis, or increased opportunities for infection, reported infection has become more widespread.

Even in areas of St. Lucia with moderately high prevalences of the schistosomal infection, however, very few of the individuals having the infection sustain medical symptomatology specifically attributable to schistosomiasis. In part, this may be due to the nature of the species (*S. mansoni*) found on St. Lucia. As Jordan and Webbe have noted: "The established *S. mansoni* infection may not give rise to symptoms, or if present they may not be severe" [74, p. 88]. But another factor may be the apparently recent development—hence generally low intensity of infection levels—of schistosomiasis on St. Lucia.

Our empirical work, as described in chapter 5 and its appendices, relates to individuals *infected* with schistosomiasis and other parasitic diseases, as revealed by the presence of ova in fecal specimens. In some of our studies our data *do* include certain symptomatological variables—enlargement of liver and/or spleen, lowered hemoglobin levels, and abdominal complaints. Though these are believed to be caused by severe schistosome infections, the symptoms are not highly specific to schistosomiasis; further the number of persons displaying the strongest symptoms, liver and/or spleen enlargement, in our studies were quite small relative to the number excreting schistosome ova. Thus, most parasite-infected persons may not have a *disease* in the medical sense that a disease is "a definite morbid process having a characteristic train of symptoms . . ." [68]. It may be that in only a small proportion of persons infected with schistosomiasis does the infection progress to an extreme level at which clinical symptoms appear. On the other hand it may be the case that a pathogenic progression occurs such that the persons who are not "sick" from the infection at one point in time will become sick at a later date. We simply cannot be sure.

As already noted in chapter 3, St. Lucia fits the typical case of less-developed countries where the prevalence of schistosomiasis is highest. It has a low average income per head, is heavily dependent on export agriculture, and its crop structure, island geography and terrain, and heavy annual rainfall all contribute to the conditions that make schistosomiasis so difficult to eradicate. Moreover, the prevailing low level of health and nutrition in the island are additional and extenuating complications. Four other parasitic diseases, for example, are commonly found in St. Lucia, though the extent of their island-wide prevalence is not known. It will turn out that the existence of these other parasites in the test population of this study will greatly complicate the analysis with respect to schistosomiasis. On the other hand, the importance of these parasites in St. Lucia and their world-wide importance suggest that a closer examination of the four parasites is worthwhile.

Other Parasites in St. Lucia

These four other parasites (all intestinal nematodes) are: *Ascaris, Trichuris*, hookworm, and *Strongyloides*. *Ascaris* is thought to be one of the most prevalent of all of man's parasites. *Trichuris* is one of the most harmful parasites which infect children. These two parasites frequently appear together. Both require no intermediate host, as does the parasite causing schistosomiasis, and both depend on fecal contamination of the environment for their origin. Though they are believed to have less serious effects on the human body than schistosomiasis, both parasites can cause great discomfort and inconvenience. Hookworm, of course, is a well-known parasite whose mode of transmission again requires contact of human skin with feces-contaminated soil. *Strongyloides* is one of the most versatile parasites known and can live indefinitely in warm, moist, fecally polluted soil [73].

The presence of these four additional parasites in St. Lucia reinforces what has been noted earlier: the interconnection between low levels of health and low average income per head. These four parasites present health problems not only in St. Lucia but in the rest of the less-developed world. It has been estimated, for example, that there are some 460 million infections of hookworm [72, p. 436]. The disease caused by *Ascaris* also has a world-wide distribution, with incidences in parts of the Far East reported at 90 percent or more [72, p. 430]. The helminthic diseases are intertwined with poor sanitation, poverty, and the basic life-style of people accustomed to barely managing to survive in a hostile natural environment. While our principal focus in this study is schistosomiasis, we shall not ignore these other helminths.

Benefits From Schistosomiasis Eradication

Schistosomiasis is peculiarly a fitting test for the application of economic analysis to health and development problems: the principal observed effect that the disease is alleged to have is malaise and lethargy, with the strong implication that human performance, whether it be the fertility potential of women, the mortality experience among women and men, the performance of children in school, or the productivity of workers in the labor force, is affected adversely by moderate levels of infection of the disease, and surely by chronically intensive levels of infection. Infection rates do vary widely, and there is still not enough evidence to differentiate intensity levels of infection within humans across countries and across species. Nonetheless, the presumed economic benefits, stemming from control and/or eradication are asserted by many authorities to be large. As noted in chapter 2 one authority has predicted that the increase in schistosomiasis created by the Aswan High Dam in Egypt will cancel any economic benefits that the dam may yield. Field studies in Iran, the Philippines, Japan, and Puerto Rico have also suggested that elimination of the disease would produce extensive net benefits, particularly with respect to the productivity of workers in agriculture, and thus, by implication, net benefits in total agricultural output [96] [105] [137] [157].

All of these studies have argued for extensive net benefits from eradication on the evidence of the high rates of *prevalence* of the disease, but
with scant evidence regarding the relationship between prevalence, on the
one hand, and disease effects, on the other.

A few studies have focused directly on the working population and have
compared worker performance before and after infection. A number of
studies have also examined school performance of infected and noninfected children, principally because many studies, showing the age
distribution of prevalence rates, revealed higher prevalence rates for
school-age children than for adults.

While the economic and social losses from schistosomiasis may well be
large, the truth is that sufficient data to test this proposition have thus
far not been available. Nonetheless, even if the "losses" turn out to be
small or negligible, from the point of view of control, it may still be useful to devote resources to a target disease *if* the effects of the control
program go beyond that disease. For example, one control technique for
reducing the rate of schistosomiasis infection is to install a central water-
supply system with safe water being piped to each house. The expected
result would be a reduction in individuals' contact with infested water.
In addition, however—and this is the central point being made here—
other results or by-products of the program could include (1) reductions
in infection from other, especially, water-borne diseases, and (2) reduction in the time and effort devoted by the population to fetching water
for the household, carrying clothing to streams for washing, and so forth.
The *total* benefits from a piped-clean-water system would thus be the
summation of these benefits and the benefits from reduced schistosomiasis
infection (however large or small these benefits might be). It is, after all,
such total benefits that should be compared with program costs as a basis
for resource-allocation decisions, not solely the benefits from control of
the target disease.

We report next on our quantitative studies of the effects of schistosomiasis and other parasitic diseases in St. Lucia.

Part II

FINDINGS
AND CONCLUSIONS

5

EFFECTS OF
SCHISTOSOMIASIS AND
OTHER PARASITIC DISEASES
IN ST. LUCIA

As can be seen from our discussion in chapter 2, estimates of the effects of schistosomiasis and other parasitic diseases have already been made by others. In large measure, these estimates have been based on what amounts to anecdotal information or have been little more than collections of simple descriptive statistics. Most have been based on impressionistic judgments or on simple statistical investigations that have failed to control for the effects of nondisease conditions or even for the effects of diseases other than the one(s) being studied.

In this chapter we will describe the extensive empirical investigations we undertook in order to carry the study of schistosomiasis and its effects beyond the realm of conjecture. The chapter not only describes our quantitative studies, however, but also presents the theoretic framework within which the data were used and the statistical analyses we employed in order to draw reasonably definitive conclusions about the effects (if any) of schistosomiasis in St. Lucia.

We mounted four separate field surveys during our enquiry. The first was a questionnaire administered to households in two St. Lucian valleys —Cul-de-Sac and Roseau. The second was an island-wide survey of schoolchildren aged thirteen to fourteen. The third was an occupational survey (in addition to the household survey) taken of workers employed by one of the largest banana-growing estates on St. Lucia. Finally, an on-the-job interview was given to a group of women working in an urban light-industry plant, with additional information on their work behavior being obtained from the plant manager.[1] Tests for the presence of schistosomes and other parasites were administered in connection with each of the surveys mentioned above, and in addition local birth and death records over a five-year period were collected and tabulated.

With this large and diverse data base to work with, we undertook several separate statistical analyses. In each study our intent was the same—to advance the understanding of the quantitative impact of parasitic diseases themselves, and also to improve on the theoretical framework within which such estimates are made for any disease and any region. Generally speaking, our statistical testing consisted of multiple regression analyses, using various functional forms and various specifications of variables to test specified hypotheses.

Separate studies were carried out to test the effects of schistosomiasis on each of the following important economic magnitudes: birth and death rates, scholastic performance of schoolchildren, rural labor productivity, and urban labor productivity.

Initially it was also planned to examine quantitatively the influence of parasitic infection on individuals' expenditure and savings behavior. The hypothesis was that infected people, and epecially those who were most severely infected, would tend to exhibit less future-oriented behavior; thus, they would save less, including spending less on relatively long-lived consumer durable goods, than would their less-infected counterparts who were similar in age, schooling-level, income, and so on. A survey instrument was developed but ultimately not utilized. Consultation with knowledgeable persons in St. Lucia convinced us that the low levels of population sophistication would not contribute to obtaining meaningful responses to questions regarding income, expenditure patterns, and saving behavior. In addition, our own field-testing indicated that the interviews were extremely time-consuming and, hence, costly, and the accuracy of findings was questionable. Perhaps such a study will be feasible, at reasonable cost, in some other region at some other time.

The methods used, the functional forms, and the tabulated results are fully discussed in the statistical appendices to this book. Any reader who wants to go further into the methodology employed and the detailed statistics compiled is urged to examine these appendices. Here the discussion will be limited to a specification of the hypotheses tested, a listing of the dependent and independent variables used, and a description of the results obtained.

1. Appendix F presents information regarding the representativeness of each of our bodies of survey data.

The Data

DEMOGRAPHIC DATA

The data which form the basis for the demographic analysis come from a household survey undertaken in the Cul-de-Sac and Roseau valleys. (This and other survey instruments used are included in Appendix A.) In Roseau, some 2,996 persons were surveyed, while 4,808 persons were surveyed in the Cul-de-Sac valley. These people resided, respectively, in 588 and 983 houses, which constituted 74.4 percent and 92.7 percent of the total number of houses in each valley.[2] The total of 7,804 rural persons covered in the two surveys amounted to more than 7 percent of the *total* population of St. Lucia, approximately 110,000 in 1967, and about 13 percent of the *rural* population. In addition to the variety of questions which we asked of respondents, a stool specimen was requested from each household member by a Research and Control Department parasitological survey team, and was actually obtained for 4,668 persons, a response rate of 60 percent. The stools were tested for the presence of schistosomiasis, and hookworm, *Ascaris*, *Trichuris*, and *Strongyloides* infections.[3]

The information on deaths collected in the household survey is unfortunately quite imperfect. Not only are deaths grossly underreported by the household respondents—the death rate per year was found to be about 4/1000 whereas the death rate for St. Lucia as a whole was officially reported to be between 7/1000 and 12/1000 in the late 1960s—but biases by sex (the male-female ratio is 4/1) are clearly apparent.[4] For this reason, official death records were also collected and tabulated for each of the areas within the two valleys for the five-year period 1964–1968.

EDUCATION DATA

In addition to the household survey and the collection of death records, an island-wide school survey of thirteen- to fourteen-year-olds was under-

2. The greater response rate in Cul-de-Sac resulted from repeated visits to houses in which no one was present when the interviewer came to the house; in Roseau only one visit was made to each house. For a discussion of why this procedure does not constitute a methodological bias, see Appendix F.

3. Qualitative stool examination for the presence of *S. mansoni*, hookworm, *Ascaris*, *Trichuris*, and *Strongyloides* ova was done according to the sedimentation-concentration technique described by E. C. Faust [87, pp. 591–592].

4. There is no easy explanation for the apparent underreporting of deaths. One possible source of error may have resulted from the nature of the question asked in the survey: "Have there been any deaths in this household in the last two years?" Since households frequently dissolve upon the death of a member, the questionnaire may have missed some of the deaths that occurred.

taken. Since the prevalence of schistosomiasis seems to "peak" around that age cohort, we decided that such an age stratification would best assure us of drawing an adequate sample of schistosomiasis sufferers and of achieving some variation in intensity levels. Moreover, given the fact that children are commonly subject to repeated re-infection with schistosomiasis while they play in infested streams and ponds, and given the cumulative effects of repeated re-infection with schistosomiasis (chapter 4), the thirteen- to fourteen-year-olds are likely to display a sizable impact of that disease. Even greater effects might be postulated for somewhat older children, but the high dropout rate at ages beyond fourteen led us to favor the thirteen to fourteen age group.

All schools having pupils in grades Standard 6 and Form 2, both of which contain the thirteen- to fourteen-year-olds, were visited—forty-five schools in all—and the child sitting in every ninth occupied seat was selected for the sample. Grades Standard 6 and Form 2 both represent the ninth year of formal education, and so the children in those grades are equivalent in age and amount of prior schooling. Standard 6 is found in most primary schools and is usually the terminal year for children in the senior cycle of the primary school. Form 2, on the other hand, is the second grade of the secondary level and represents an early stage in the training of youths pursuing an advanced program. Thus, there is a priori reason to believe that students in Standard 6 and Form 2 differ systematically in their motivations, aspirations, and family backgrounds. In our empirical analysis we take account of these differences, but on an individual student basis rather than on a school-by-school basis. Finally, Standard 6 is the last grade before which the attrition rate is critical, and in almost all areas of the island there are no opportunities to go beyond it.

Location of school was used as a proxy for a pupil's residence, and locations were categorized as follows: Castries (the capital and principal city), other urban, and rural. Data on a pupil's socio-economic status—as indicated by father's occupation and father's education—on sources of water, and on his or her beliefs about the nature and causes of disease were derived from responses to a questionnaire (see Appendix A). Scores on the Nelson Reading Test for grades 3–9 were used as the index of scholastic performance [216]. The Nelson Reading Test, although standardized for pupils in the United States, was judged by several St. Lucian school authorities to be sufficiently free of (North American) cultural bias for our purposes and to conform to the comprehension level of normal St. Lucian Standard 6 and Form 2 schoolchildren. To minimize bias arising from differences in classroom conditions, and particularly in teachers' behavior, the survey instruments were administered uniformly

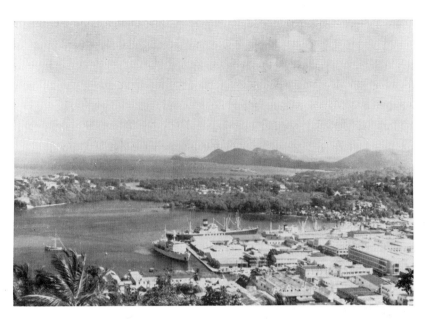

Inner harbor and downtown area of St. Lucia's capital city, Castries

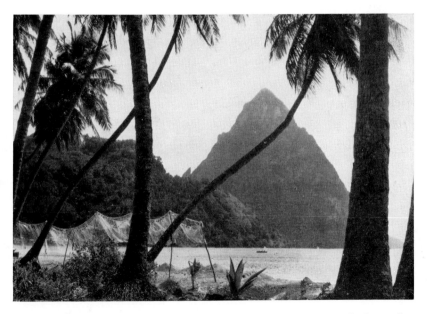

View near town of Soufriere: *foreground*—fishermen's nets drying; *background*—Petit Piton, a volcanic dome

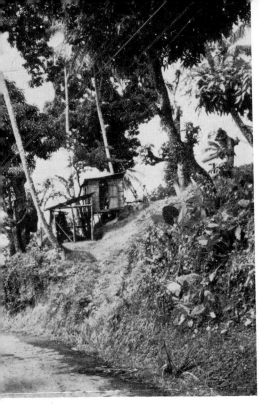

Common rural St. Lucian household

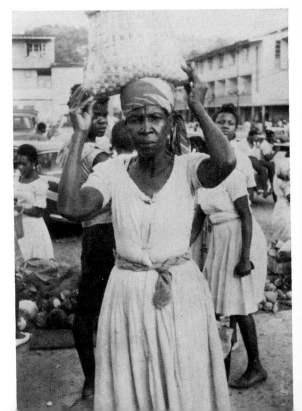

Woman carrying purchases from
Castries market

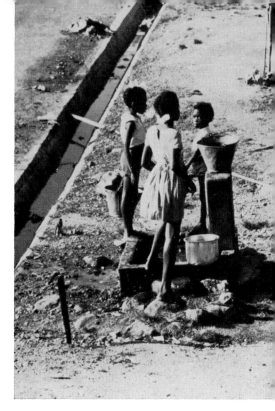

Getting water from one of the few community taps

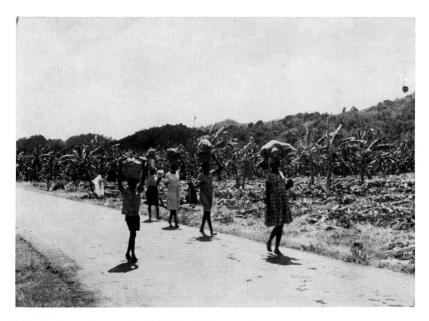

"Heading" supplies on the Cul-de-Sac Valley road

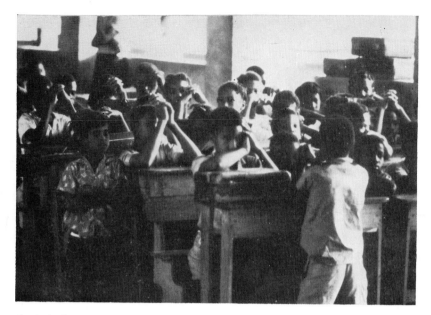

A rural classroom

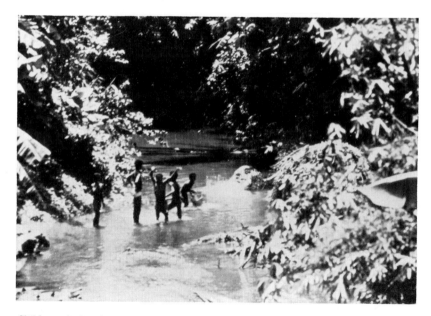

Children playing in a stream where schistosomiasis transmission probably occurs

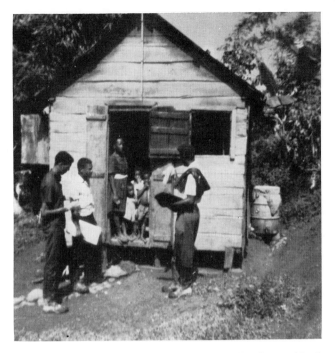

A Roseau Valley household being interviewed by the combined parasitological and economic survey teams

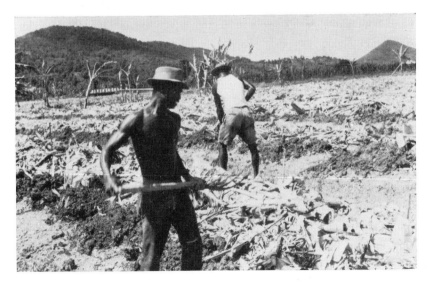

Workers on the Geest banana estate at Cul-de-Sac, preparing a field for replanting

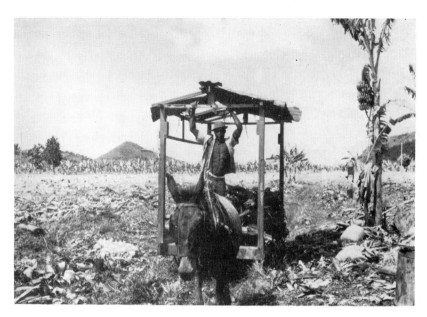

Banana "seed" being brought to a field by rail carriage

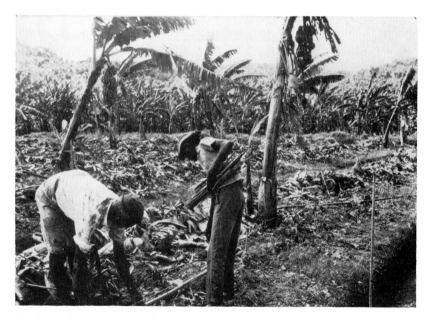

Placing stakes at measured distances to indicate where seed should be planted

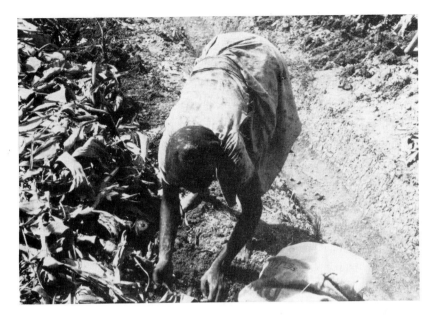

Planting the seed

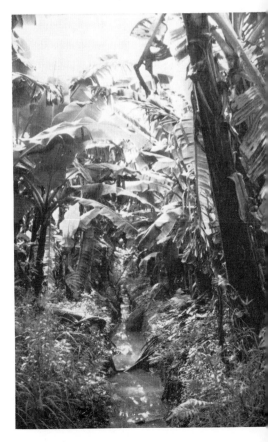

Mature banana field—these drainage ditches
between rows are a potential source of
schistosomiasis transmission

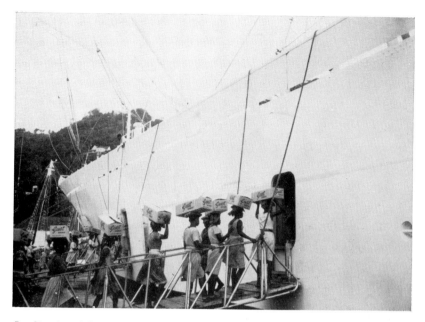

Loading boxed bananas on a Geest ship at Castries

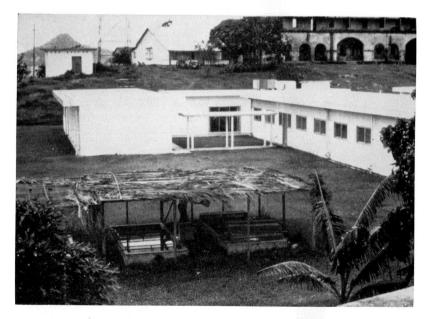

Research and Control Department: The Rockefeller Foundation-supported schisto-somiasis research station near Castries in all schools by a trained bilingual (English- and patois-speaking) native St. Lucian. This school sample yielded 162 pupils, of which 158 furnished stools that were tested for infection with schistosomes and the other four parasites.

We also used another body of school data, which had been obtained shortly prior to our study, and which was made available by the Research and Control Department. This consisted of a collection of information on schoolchildren in a rural area of high schistosomiasis prevalence—Babonneau. Two hundred and sixty-seven children generally aged nine to fourteen in five class grades (Standards 2–6) were studied in regard to the effects of schistosomiasis on the pupils' (1) weight, (2) height, (3) class rank, and (4) attendance at school. The effects of the *intensity* of schistosomiasis infection was tested with the use of a quantitative examination of the schistosome eggs per gram of stool.[5] In addition, data on three other parasites—hookworm, *Ascaris,* and *Trichuris,* but not *Strongyloides* —were available to us, as were data on age and sex. In the Babonneau study there were no data on socio-economic characteristics of individual students.

AGRICULTURAL LABOR-PRODUCTIVITY DATA

For the agricultural labor-productivity study, we collected data for 466 men and women. The data covered daily physical output and daily earnings for workers performing eight different piece-rate, or "task," jobs, as well as daily attendance and earnings information for "day" (nonpiece work) labor, over the eighteen-month period, January 1, 1966, through June 30, 1967. A supplementary questionnaire, in addition to the household survey mentioned above, was also administered to these 466 people to get more detailed information on their habitual work patterns. (A copy of the supplementary questionnaire is in Appendix A.)

We also collected health information about these particular workers— specifically: (1) the presence or absence of schistosomiasis and each of the four parasites enumerated above; (2) a quantitative examination of excreted schistosome ova for many of those persons having schistoso-

5. The quantitative stool examination for *S. mansoni* ova employed the filtration-staining technique, using 5 ml. of stool (measured by displacement) in 50 ml. of water, as described by D. R. Bell [85].

While the host load of schistosome worms and the number of schistosome eggs *retained* in body tissues are the actual determinants of intensity, counting *excreted* eggs is considered the most practical measure of intensity [127, p. 26] [156, p. 9]. Some doubts have been cast, however, on the relevance of the egg count. For example, M. Farooq et al. found no relationship between egg output and the severity of clinical symptoms for *S. mansoni* infections in Egypt [86]. Peter Jordan, on the other hand, believes egg-counting to be a useful diagnostic tool [89] [143].

miasis; and (3) information on the presence and degree of liver and spleen enlargement and on low hemoglobin count—all of which are symptoms of severe cases of schistosomiasis, though also of severe cases of other diseases. Because we lack information about health conditions and diseases other than these, we are assuming, in effect, that any other factors that affect labor productivity are randomly distributed in the population sample tested.

Although our total sample size was 466 individuals, complete information was not available for each individual. At least one stool examination for the presence of schistosome ova was performed for every one of the 466, but because a person who has schistosomiasis may not pass eggs in each stool, multiple tests were performed to the extent possible. Of the 466 persons, 153 were tested only once, and for this group the danger of a "false negative," that is, not finding schistosomiasis when the person actually has it, is greatest; 313 persons were tested at least twice, and 150 were tested three or four times. Since complete survey information was not obtained for all in the sample, however, the actual sample size used in each of our analyses was further limited, to 126 or less (66 males and 60 females).

URBAN LABOR-PRODUCTIVITY DATA

Lastly, in order to learn something about the effects of parasites on the productivity of urban workers, we collected data on 114 women who worked for Dimensions, Ltd., for the period May 1968 to July 1969. The following personal information was obtained by interview on the job: age, years of schooling, marital status ("living with a man"—a common answer—was counted as "married"), number of dependents, and place of residence (this was later coded as urban, semi-urban, or rural). Data on attendance, absenteeism, physical productivity, and weekly earnings for each worker were obtained from the plant manager. Parasitic-infection information was obtained from laboratory examination of a stool specimen provided by the worker.

The Analyses and Results

The findings of each of our six statistical studies are summarized separately below. The natality and mortality studies are discussed in greater detail in Appendix B. The detailed analyses of the two bodies of data on academic achievement of schoolchildren will be found in Appendix C. And the details of the rural and urban labor-productivity studies are in Appendix D.

NATALITY

A priori, there appears to be no *direct* connection between schistoso-miasis and the biological processes associated with conception or child-bearing. Thus it might be expected that the birth rate is independent of the presence or severity of schistosomiasis. On the other hand, in those severe cases in which schistosomiasis diminishes the effectiveness of the liver, spleen, and intestines, thereby negatively affecting general health, it might affect both the ability to conceive and the ability to bring a child to term. Furthermore, as is the case with all parasitic diseases, not only are the schistosome parasites an irritant to the biological system, but they also divert a portion of the nutrient value of foods and fluids away from other biological processes, including that of childbearing. In ad-dition, schistosomiasis seems likely to retard the birth rate since both the probability of marrying and the frequency of sexual relations are likely to be influenced by an individual's general state of health. We therefore postulated that schistosomiasis and the four other parasitic dis-eases depress the natality or birth rate.[6]

Several possible hypotheses describe the specific relationship between disease and the birth rate. In this study we explored only two: an inter-action model and an additive model. The interaction model is one which considers the impact on the birth rate of parasitic diseases working in combination as well as singly. This formulation admits the possibility that the impact on births of combinations of diseases may be different from the simple additive impacts of the individual diseases. The second formu-lation, the additive model, assumes that the impact of combinations of diseases is simply the summation of the impact of the individual diseases. In both formulations of the determinants of the birth rate we controlled not only for the presence of each of the five parasites but also for the woman's age and education.

The statistical results using the interaction model yielded the expected negative relationships between the birth rate, on the one hand, and age and education, on the other. However, the hypothesis concerning a nega-tive effect of parasitic diseases on the birth rate was not supported (see Table B.2). In the Cul-de-Sac valley, for example, schistosomiasis was found to have a significant *positive* association with births. (The inter-pretation that the disease *causes* an increased birth rate is one that may not seem plausible; however, it is possible that persons who suffer from disease may turn more to sexual gratification.) In the two valleys, only

6. An interesting hypothesis, which should be investigated in future studies, is that parasites so weaken mothers that they bear sickly children, who, in turn, have high subsequent infant and child mortality. This was suggested by Peter Newman.

four of the disease interaction terms were significant, and in each of these cases, the sign was also positive rather than the expected negative (see Table B.2). Finally, in no case did we find a significant effect for the same combination of diseases for both Cul-de-Sac and Roseau.

This might lead us to reject the four significant interaction terms as spurious. But in all four combinations of diseases that were significant, *Ascaris* is the only common element. Since it is basically a garden parasite, the statistical findings may be identifying the probability of new mothers contracting the disease caused by *Ascaris* rather than its impact on the birth rate. This might be the case if new mothers were more likely than others to be out-of-doors. Identifying the direction of causation remains an unsolved problem, and indeed we cannot dismiss the possibility that causation runs in two directions—from birth rate to disease as well as from disease to birth rate. (An investigation of the possibility of reverse causation for schistosomiasis and natality is described in Appendix B.)

The additive model—in which the impact of each disease on the birth rate is assumed to be the summation of the individual impacts of each disease—was next tested, and several conclusions emerged from this analysis. Again we found no evidence that schistosomiasis or the *Trichuris* or hookworm parasites exert a significant negative impact on the birth rate (see Table B.3). *Strongyloides*, however, was shown to have a significant and negative impact on births in both valleys, and *Ascaris* again was found to be associated with a significant *positive* impact on the birth rate in one valley, Cul-de-Sac. The estimated parameter for *Strongyloides* was almost identical in each of the two populations. While *Strongyloides* has not been linked directly with the reproductive system, indirect connections do exist. This parasite does attack the intestines by burrowing into the mucosa of the intestinal walls. This can cause periods of extreme constipation, diarrhea, and vomiting, which can have an adverse effect on a pregnant woman's ability to bring a fetus to term.[7]

Even though the primary focus in this study is schistosomiasis, the possible impact of *Strongyloides* on the birth rate is noteworthy. Since certain types of schistosomiasis-control programs (e.g., latrine construction) are likely to reduce the prevalence of other parasitic diseases, including that caused by *Strongyloides*, the impact of these other parasites is important in evaluating control programs for schistosomiasis.

We obtained a measure of the impact of *Strongyloides* infection on

7. There is some doubt, however, whether the low-intensity infection levels of *Strongyloides* found in St. Lucia are likely to cause the described symptomatic effects.

births by estimating, for those sixty-three women who had it, the number of births that had been prevented by the infection. During a two-year period, 10.6 births were predicted for the sixty-three women carrying the *Strongyloides* parasite; a similar calculation assuming the absence of this parasite yielded a prediction of 36.0 births. Thus, elimination of *Strongyloides* is estimated to increase the birth rate for those mothers infected with the disease by about 240 percent. On the other hand, since only a small fraction of the total female population (about 10 percent) was infected with *Strongyloides* parasites, the impact of the disease's elimination would result in a much smaller, though still substantial, increase in the aggregate birth rate—about 16 percent.[8]

These results illustrate the importance of taking into account the many linkages between health and demographic change. Thus, when considering the impact of one disease—schistosomiasis—on economic and social behavior, it is necessary to consider not only the direct linkages of this particular disease to various economic and demographic variables, but also the connections between schistosomiasis and other diseases, together with the impact of those other diseases on behavior. The above results, showing a marked increase in the birth rate likely to result indirectly from a particular type of schistosomiasis-control program—where a side-effect is a reduction in the incidence of *Strongyloides*—illustrate well the necessity of a comprehensive approach to the analysis of disease, demographic change, and economic growth.

MORTALITY

The basic hypothesis to be tested in this section is that schistosomiasis and other parasitic diseases decrease an individual's life expectancy—or, in other words, increase the death rate.

The medical literature provides almost no solid evidence concerning the magnitude of the mortality impact of schistosomiasis, although speculations are abundant [149] [156, p. 44] [75] [137, p. 105] [76] [133]. At the one extreme, a major study of schistosomiasis by the WHO concludes that "Normally, bilharziasis [schistosomiasis] neither kills nor incapacitates completely . . ." [76]. At the other extreme, studies have noted "Up to 12 percent of the people autopsied after dying in hospitals in parts of South America died of the consequences of schistosome infection" [156], and ". . . death was attributed to the infection in 8.2 percent of subjects by Koppisch (1940–41)" [137]. A careful review of

---

8. This figure was derived by dividing the increase in births (36.0 − 10.6) due to an eradication of *Strongyloides* by the total number of births actually recorded in Cul-de-Sac and Roseau valleys during the period of this study.

the literature reveals, however, that most of the "evidence" on the mortality impact of schistosomiasis is conjectural; little, if any, is based on acceptable statistical or scientific grounds. That evidence which does exist is typically obtained from an identification of the "immediate" cause of death as revealed by autopsy.

We are not concerned, however, with the immediate or even the "primary" cause of death. Indeed, it is probable that schistosomiasis, like many other diseases, exerts its mortality effect not by acting as the immediate cause of death, but rather by affecting the individual's general state of health; the latter, in turn, influencing the length of life. Respiratory diseases, and in particular tuberculosis and pneumonia, rank high as "causes" of death throughout much of the tropics. But resistance to these diseases is related to the general health of the individual, which, in turn, is believed to be affected directly by the individual's parasitological history. Thus, while schistosomiasis and other parasitic diseases may not appear in autopsies or other observations as a frequent "cause" of death, their mortality impact might nevertheless be considerable. It is this broader conception of the determinants of death which forms the basis of our analysis.

The mortality effect of disease can be explored at the individual level (probability of death) or at the group level (the death rate). The mortality data from the household survey proved to be of such poor quality, however, that we could not pursue the former tactic and were restricted to death-rate statistics.

The findings are again surprising. None of the independent variables (age, sex, disease prevalence) exerted a significant impact on death rates, regardless of which regression form was used (see Table B.5). A seriously constraining factor in the statistical analysis is the limited number of subgroup observations and, hence, degrees of freedom. For this reason, our findings are certainly not a definitive rejection of the hypothesis that death rates in St. Lucia are substantially affected by parasitic infections.

ACADEMIC PERFORMANCE

Several previous attempts have been made in other regions of the world to determine whether schistosomiasis has a significant impact on schoolchildren's performance. Taken collectively, these investigations have yielded inconclusive results, both because the findings have conflicted and because they have not embodied adequate controls in regard to other health factors or to nonhealth factors likely to influence schoolchildren's performance—including their socio-economic and ethnographic backgrounds. In addition, most of these studies lacked tests of statistical significance for assessing the effects of disease. We turn now to a brief review of these studies, bearing in mind that we are covering investigations that deal with three different species of schistosomiasis and that each does not necessarily have the same impact on the children's performance.

Among the earliest efforts to ascertain a relationship between schistosomiasis and achievement in school was a study in Rhodesia (formerly Southern Rhodesia) of children in two European-type boys' secondary schools, one "academic" and the other "modern" [84].[9] Boys in the academic school, where the prevalence rate of schistosomiasis (*S. haematobium*) was significantly lower, performed better in end-of-term examinations than did the boys in the modern school. The proportions of pupils coming from urban and rural areas were about the same in both schools, which led the investigators to assume sampling comparability between the two groups and to conclude that all of the differential in scholastic achievement was attributable to the difference in the prevalence rates of schistosomiasis. That conclusion is questionable, however, in view of the higher scholastic standards for admission ordinarily attributed to the academic secondary schools.

Similarly, in South Africa it was stated that the symptoms of schistosomiasis in schoolchildren appeared to be "forgetfulness, indifference to punishment, apparent laziness and disinclination to mental exertion combined with a sometimes very marked nervous irritability, obstreperousness and mental fatigue" [145]. These symptoms apparently tended to "disappear completely" upon treatment of the disease with an antimony preparation. The findings of that study, however, were based exclusively on personal impression and the subjective reports of schoolteachers; no systematic attempt was made to match schistosomiasis sufferers with nonsufferers in assessing effects of the disease.

On the other hand, a later investigation in Rhodesia found that schoolchildren with schistosomiasis (*S. haematobium*) actually performed better than did uninfected pupils [148]. In a primary school with a schistosomiasis-prevalence rate of 50 percent, most of the infected children ranked scholastically in the top half of their class and most of the students who failed the end-of-term examination were free of disease. Nevertheless, in the absence of tests for statistical significance or adequate experimental controls, these findings, too, are questionable.

In a virtual replication of the Rhodesian study, this time among Sukuma

9. An "academic" secondary school offers a college preparatory program. A "modern" secondary school offers a mixture of college preparatory and vocational subjects and is generally less selective in its admission of pupils than the "academic" secondary school.

schoolchildren in Tanzania (formerly Tanganyika), no association was found between the prevalence of schistosomiasis and scholastic performance [153]. Interestingly, these findings were not consistent with the subjective impressions of headmasters, who were convinced that schistosomiasis had an adverse effect on their pupils' schoolwork.

Additional evidence to suggest that schistosomiasis (*S. haematobium*) has no harmful effect on academic performance derives from another study in Tanzania [144]. In three out of the four school grades surveyed, infected children actually had higher examination scores than did uninfected pupils, though whether the differences were statistically significant was not reported.

Although the relationship between schistosomiasis and scholastic performance is unclear, available evidence suggests that that disease can retard physical development. In a study of Egyptian children it was shown that, given an absence of other pathological and nutritional disturbances, schistosomiasis (*S. haematobium* and *S. mansoni* were both present) stunted height and otherwise delayed skeletal maturation [151]. Similarly, a report on Tanzanian pupils disclosed that the mean weight and mean height of children with schistosomiasis (*S. mansoni*) were lower than for pupils not found infected with that parasite, and these results were consistent in all four grades studied. Moreover, the exercise tolerance of a group infected with schistosomiasis (*S. haematobium*) was lower than for the uninfected group, though the difference was reported as being not statistically significant. (The level of significance, however, was not reported [144].)

If schistosomiasis does influence physical maturation, and if academic performance is affected by physical development [218] [219] [227]—a matter that is not clear—we would expect to find that schistosomiasis does retard academic performance. The conflicting findings of the studies noted above, however, may be partly ascribable to the inadequate controls for such social and economic variables as parental occupation and education and urban-rural differences. One of the studies in Tanzania surveyed children mainly from rural areas, and the sample was selective in that the pupils were required to have passed a test before enrolling in the school [235] [144]. The other study in Tanzania and those in Rhodesia and South Africa similarly failed to account for differences in family backgrounds (socio-economic status) or for uban-rural differences among schoolchildren [84] [145] [153]. Yet, omission of such factors can bias the findings; children of parents with relatively low socio-economic status or from rural areas may be more likely to have schistosomiasis, so that any differences in achievement may derive as much or more from family background than children's health characteristics.

Such background factors, after all, have been found to influence academic performance. A national study of schoolchildren in the United States found that achievement in reading dramatically differentiated pupils in urban schools of different socio-economic levels [204].[10] Similarly, in an international study of achievement in mathematics, it was shown that students with parents in the highest occupational groups scored higher than students with parents in the lowest occupational groups in eight out of nine countries for which information was available [207]. Other studies have rather consistently found strong correlations between an individual pupil's social class level and many aspects of his school career [190] [193] [194] [199] [27] [202] [205] [223] [225] [226].

Using data from our island-wide survey described above, we hypothesized the following: that pupil's achievement scores would be positively affected by urban residence, especially residence in Castries (the capital), and by father's socio-economic status, including father's education and occupation. On the other hand, we expected to find that achievement scores would be negatively affected by disease infection, by the use of hazardous sources of water (to drink, bathe in, and launder in), and by lack of knowledge of germ theory. We then used data on the Babonneau school located in a high prevalence area (described above) to test the above hypotheses. Our hypothesis, again, was that schistosomiasis, alone or in combination with other parasitic diseases, exerts a *negative* effect on the child's vitality and physical condition. Thus, we expected to find from the Babonneau data that the presence of parasitic infection would be associated with low weight of child, low height, low rank in class, and high absenteeism.

In fact, we found that the effects of the parasitic infections were not significant, either in regard to pupil's academic performance, for the island as a whole (see Tables C.6 and C.7), or in relation to schoolchildren's weight or class rank in the Babonneau, high-schistosomiasis-prevalence area. (See Appendix C for details.) Schistosomiasis was significantly related (at the .05 level) to absenteeism among pupils attending school in the endemic rural area serviced by the Babonneau School, but in the direction *opposite* to our prior expectation—children with that disease were absent *less* than other children (see Table C.12). One might speculate that this finding results from the fact that absenteeism—especially in the rural areas—is often due to the demand on children to work in the fields, especially on days when bananas are harvested. Infected children may be too sick or weak to work efficiently in the

10. Parental occupation, income, and education were used as indicators of socio-economic status.

fields, but healthy enough to attend—and perform about equally well in (as indicated by our findings)—school. Even when schistosomiasis and other diseases work in combination, there is only weak evidence of any tendency to increase absences (see Tables C.12 and C.15).

Whatever the explanation, however, the finding that children with schistosomiasis, *ceteris paribus*, are absent significantly *less* from school than students without it does not confirm the initial hypothesis that the disease *increases* absenteeism from school. And, in general, our findings with respect to the barely significant relationship between schistosomal infection and children's height, and the lack of significant relationships between schistosomal infection and the other dependent variables—weight, and especially class rank—also do not confirm the hypotheses of adverse effects.

RURAL LABOR PRODUCTIVITY

Our main hypothesis in this part of the empirical analysis was that schistosomiasis and other parasitic diseases debilitate their victims and thereby diminish productive potential. By "productive potential" we mean the worker's productivity capacity, for a given number of hours worked and with a given stock and quality of capital, land, and other complementary resources.

It is difficult to measure *potential* productivity; hence, we examined first the hypothesis that the parasitic infections cut *actual* productivity as measured by actual labor market earnings. Specifically, we studied the empirical relationship between earnings per week—as a measure of productivity—and the presence of schistosomiasis and each of the other four parasitic infections, acting singly and in combination.

Actual productivity for any worker, as measured by his weekly earnings, is a function of two variables, each of which we examined separately. First, weekly earnings depend upon the type of work he performs and on his productivity at that work. Second, weekly earnings depend on the number of days worked per week.

The fact that a worker can be expected to adjust to any debilitating effects of disease by shifting to work that is less demanding physically or may alter the amount of time worked confounds the attempt to assess the effects of disease on productive *potential*. Debilitation may be thought of as a change in relative prices confronting a worker, or specifically, as a change in relative wages he can earn at various types of work and at work versus leisure. A drop in the ill worker's productive potential will thus tend to bring about changes (income and substitution effects) in both the type of work performed and the amount of time worked per week. As a result, in order to understand better the effects of disease on productive potential, it is necessary to examine not only the effects on total weekly earnings but also the workers' adjustments in the type and amount of work performed.

Therefore, in addition to testing our main hypothesis (1) that disease leads to reduced earnings, we also tested three hypotheses that underlie it: "ill" workers, as gauged by the presence of parasites in their bodies,[11] work at jobs that are physically less demanding (hypothesis 2); they are less productive per day worked on any given type of work (hypothesis 3); and they work fewer days per week (hypothesis 4).[12]

Hypothesis 1 (disease infection leads to reduced weekly earnings) was tested with the body of data collected from the Geest agricultural workers. The dependent variable in our regression models was earnings per week and the independent variables included tests for presence or absence of each parasite in a given person and the person's age, education, housing circumstances, and so on (see Tables D.2 and D.3). The results showed that only one parasitic variable was significant—and that one, *Strongyloides*, was statistically significant only for females. With this one exception, we failed to find support for the hypothesis that schistosomiasis or any of the other parasitic diseases, individually, depress actual productivity as reflected by weekly earnings. On the other hand, in one regression we found that although no individual disease had a significant negative effect, the total effect on weekly earnings of the *entire group* of parasitic infections was significantly negative.

Hypothesis 2 (ill workers work at physically less-demanding jobs) was then tested.

The individual worker on the Geest estate can, to a considerable extent, decide for himself whether to do "task" work (for which piece rates are paid) or "day" work. Although task work is physically more demanding than day work, a highly productive worker can earn considerably more per day on a task job; consequently this type of work generally is regarded as highly desirable. The amount of task work available is limited, but each worker is given essentially the same opportunity by the overseers to choose task work. Thus, since each worker could choose to do day work or task work, we used the distinction between task work and day

11. Note that the word "ill" is used here only to indicate infection; infected persons are not necessarily "ill" in the sense of manifesting symptoms of disease.

12. Days per week—rather than days per month or per year—were selected as the dependent variable in testing the relationship between illnesses and labor supply because medical examinations and interviews suggested that most of any effects of disease on the labor supply would manifest themselves in this variable. Factors difficult to quantify are also likely to be significant in accounting for differences in weeks worked per month or year.

work as equivalent to the choice between more-demanding and less-demanding work. The dependent variable used in our test of Hypothesis 2 was the proportion of days of task work to total days worked for each individual,[13] and the independent variables were the same as used in testing hypothesis 1 (see Table D.4).

Once again, our hypothesis was not supported. None of the diseases or other variables was significant in explaining the observed variation among workers in the percentage of task work performed.

Hypothesis 3 (ill workers' productivity per day is less than that of healthy workers) was tested using two of the dependent variables: earnings per day for all types of day and task work taken as a whole, and earnings per day for selected specific task jobs. The independent explanatory variables were again the same as above. These tests showed that schistosomiasis infection was indeed associated with lower daily earnings for males, and presence of *Strongyloides* was significantly related to lower earnings for females (see Table D.5). The estimated effect on earnings of being infected with schistosomiasis is a quite substanial reduction of about 80 cents (E.C.) per day, a reduction of about 30 percent from the average daily earnings of male plantation workers; the indicated effect of *Strongyloides* infection is a reduction of 31 cents per day, some 15 percent of average daily earnings by female plantation workers.

It is also notable that the amount of time spent in non-Geest work was, as expected, negatively related to the male workers' earnings per day worked at Geest. As far as the individual tasks are concerned, no very consistent pattern showed up. Schistosomiasis was even related *positively* to the daily earnings of women on one task job.[14]

These results can be regarded as providing some support for the hypothesis that schistosomiasis does act to reduce daily productivity overall. This effect does not extend over all types of task jobs, nor does presence of the infection appear to reduce the daily earnings of women. However, if earnings per day are separated into earnings from task work and earnings from jobs paying a fixed daily wage (not shown in the

13. To take account of the possibility that occasionally a worker may be pressed into task work at peak work periods and also the possibility that the effect of disease on workers' stamina is negligible over very low ranges of task work, the sample is restricted to those who have performed task work on at least ten percent of the days they have worked.

14. Presence of *Ascaris*, however, is associated with lower daily earnings for three of the six task-sex groups in Table D.6. And among males performing tasks 1 and 3, those men who also grew their own bananas earned significantly more per day working for Geest. This was as expected, and suggests that such men are among the more ambitious or more motivated to obtain money income.

appendix tables), schistosomiasis shows up as a significant variable that is negatively related to task-work earnings (but not day-work earnings) for women. On the other hand, for men, presence of schistosomiasis infection is negatively related to day-work earnings but not to task-work earnings per day. Perhaps the male workers who concentrate on day work are not as strong initially as those performing task work and, thus, are more likely to be debilitated by disease infection than are task workers.

Hypothesis 4 (infected workers have higher absentee rates than healthy ones) was tested by regressing the average number of days worked per week (during the eighteen-month period) on the same set of independent variables as above. Once again, none of the five parasitic infections was associated for males with a significantly smaller number of days worked, while for females only one parasite, *Strongyloides*, was so related (see Table D.7). For males the sign of the coefficient indicating the presence of "many eggs"—that is, intense schistosomiasis infection—was actually significantly *positive*. This finding, while surprising at first, is actually consistent with the view that workers respond to a decrease in their daily productive capacity by working more days per week in order to minimize the effect of their debility on their total weekly earnings.[15] We have already seen that schistosomiasis infection is reducing the productive *potential* of males by a rather substantial 30 percent; the process of adjustment to infection is such, however, that the reduction in productive potential is offset by an increase in the amount of time worked (Table D.7), so that actual weekly earnings (productivity) are unaffected. In short, *the cost of schistosomiasis infection for males is a reduction, not in market production and earnings, but in leisure.*

Perhaps a comparison of workers not having schistosomiasis ("healthy" workers) with those who did have it and had clinical symptoms of illness ("sick" workers) would disclose significant differences in earnings and labor effort. Our comparisons of the average daily earnings and the average days worked per week of male and of female workers in those two groups are reported and described more fully in Appendix D. We found that the healthy workers actually earned *less*, rather than more, and for males the difference was statistically significant. Regarding average days worked per week, the healthy males worked less, but the healthy females did work more; neither of these differences, however, were significant.

15. However, it is also consistent with the proposition that causality runs in the opposite direction—that persons who prefer to work longer are more likely to become infected with the disease.

URBAN LABOR PRODUCTIVITY

The bulk of workers in St. Lucia are agricultural, but a growing number are employed in the expanding urban centers. Our empirical analysis of the effects of disease on labor productivity concluded with analysis of data from a firm, Dimensions, Ltd., located in the capital city, Castries, and employing women to fold and assemble paper advertising material. Manual dexterity is required, but—or so it would appear—physical endurance is not likely to be important, by contrast with the agricultural work on the banana plantations.

For the reasons described more fully above, we hypothesized that if workers are being debilitated by schistosomiasis and other parasitic diseases, then persons with these infections would earn less (hypothesis 1), be less productive—in physical-output terms—per day worked (hypothesis 3), and be absent more from work (hypothesis 4).[16] The latter expectation, however, while quite reasonable for the hard physical work on the Geest plantations, may be inappropriate for the more sedentary tasks performed by the Dimensions, Ltd., workers while sitting before a table.

Hypothesis 1—parasitic infection is associated with lower level of weekly earnings—was tested by regressing weekly salary on the five disease variables and other independent variables similar to those in the Geest worker analyses. The results showed that none of the independent variables was significant at the .10 level, and the combination of the twelve variables explained only 12 percent of the variance in earnings (see Table D.10, column 5).

We next examined whether infected workers are less productive per day than uninfected workers (hypothesis 3). This hypothesis was tested for the dependent variable, physical output, on each of three jobs involving distinct assembly activities.

For two of the jobs, there was no evidence in support of the hypothesis that parasitic infection reduces actual productivity. For the third job, the results were somewhat different; presence of *Ascaris* was significantly associated with lower productivity, but presence of hookworm was associated with significantly *higher* levels of productivity. (The latter relationship was also found a number of times for the Geest agricultural workers.)

Finally Hypothesis 4 (infected workers are absent more) was tested by regressing the dependent variable, number of days worked as a percentage of potential work days (this was to adjust for the fact that some workers

16. Hypothesis 2—disease causes workers to shift to physically less demanding jobs—could not be tested, since the jobs performed at Dimensions, Ltd., involved a fairly uniform level of physical activity.

were hired later than others during the fourteen-month survey period), on the independent variables enumerated above. Women with urban places of residence worked significantly fewer days than did other workers (see Table D.10). This might be attributed to the generally lower family income of semi-urban and especially rural residents as compared with their urban counterparts, and the resulting greater need of the former groups to supplement the family income. The number of dependents also appeared to exert a negative impact on work attendance, suggesting that women with more dependent children took off more days from work in order to care for their children. Age was also significant, although with a negative sign, contrary to that generally found for the Geest workers. Most important, however, the negative relationship between parasite infection and work attendance stated in hypothesis 4 is certainly not confirmed by our findings: neither presence of schistosomiasis nor any of the other parasitic diseases was associated significantly with the percentage of days worked.

Summary

Our rural and urban labor-productivity results are consistent with the view that only one parasite, namely *Strongyloides*, adversely affects actual labor productivity—and then only for the female group working in agriculture.[17] Not only are weekly earnings lower for females who have this disease but daily earnings and average number of days worked per week are also lower for this group.

As far as schistosomiasis is concerned, the evidence supports the hypothesis that the daily productivity of male plantation workers, especially those working on day jobs, is decreased as a result of the infection. However, the *weekly* wages of male workers who have the infection are not lower than those who are not infected, because the infected group is absent less from the job. Whether this lower absenteeism level is the result of efforts by these workers to maintain their total income after they become ill or is due to the fact that those who work longer are more likely to contract the infection cannot be determined with our model. However, the lower *daily* productivity of those with schistosomiasis does provide direct evidence that *potential* productivity is reduced to some extent— and that was the main purpose of our inquiry. But the evidence has hardly been overwhelming, and so the conclusion that schistosomiasis reduces productive *capacity* by something near 30 percent must, therefore, be regarded as tentative.

17. The regression coefficients for this parasite for the sample of men were not significant for any of the hypotheses.

One possible explanation for our not finding stronger evidence of an adverse productivity impact from schistosomiasis is that the prevalence of the infection on a widespread basis may be of comparatively recent origin in St. Lucia. Infection may decrease productivity only after the population has been affected for several years. In a partial effort to test for this possibility, the various hypotheses were tested again using a later productivity period for Geest workers than the original January 1, 1966–June 30, 1967, interval. This later production period covered June 30, 1967, to January 1, 1969. The same parasitological data were used, however.

The results of the tests on the later period (not presented in Appendix D) support the earlier conclusion that schistosomiasis does not significantly reduce weekly productivity, as measured by earnings, either for men or women. Moreover, unlike the previous period when schistosomiasis was associated with lower *daily* earnings of men, the later interval shows no statistically significant relation. On the other hand, whereas in the first period men who were infected with schistosomiasis actually worked more days per week than those who were not, the opposite relationship holds for the later period. Conceivably, this decline in work time could indicate a growing adverse effect of schistosomiasis over time, but in view of the lack of any negative effect on daily earnings or productivity, it seems best to regard the findings for the later period as weakening the earlier findings of a negative effect of schistosomiasis on daily productivity and confirming the earlier findings that workers infected with schistosomiasis are neither absent more from work nor do they have lower weekly earnings than their noninfected counterparts.

Other than some indication that the diseases may affect daily earnings of male agricultural workers, our numerous tests have disclosed little to suggest that parasitic infections in St. Lucia are having any pronounced effects of the various types studied. There remains the possibility, though, that such effects are present but are too weak to have been detected. With this in mind, we performed another test in which all of the individual tests presented above were pooled and summarized. The objective was to determine whether these aggregated findings show any evidence of disease effects.

Appendix Table E.1 presents the results of a test in which we compared the total number of negative coefficients and the total number of positives—whether the coefficient was statistically significant or not. That is, we compared the frequency with which each disease was associated with the expected effect on any of the demographic, school-performance, or labor-productivity variables with the frequency with which an unexpected effect (regardless of magnitude or significance level) was found. The question was whether there was a statistically significant preponderance of the expected relationships.

While the full findings are in Table E.1, some of them are discussed here. For schistosomiasis there is a significant difference between the number of expected and unexpected relationships for the combined agricultural and urban labor-productivity tests (columns 7 and 8), but this preponderance of the expected relationships is largely the result of the urban labor-productivity, Dimensions, Ltd., studies (columns 4 and 5). Of the various equations, with different dependent variables, in which either the presence of schistosomiasis or the schistosome egg count appeared as an explanatory variable, we found the expected adverse relationship between schistosomiasis infection and the dependent performance variables in twenty-seven regression estimates, while only sixteen unexpected relationships were found (column 21). This preponderance, while in the expected direction, is not statistically significant.

Among the other four parasites, only one, *Ascaris,* showed a statistically significant excess of expected associations, for the various kinds of effects taken as a whole. Infection with *Ascaris* is particularly associated with significant adverse effects on labor productivity, both agricultural and urban.

The results, when pooled over all five parasitic diseases and all tests, do indicate a statistically significant preponderance of ninety-one expected effects of the diseases as compared with sixty-three unexpected effects. Schistosomiasis and *Ascaris* infection are the greatest contributors.

Overall, our pooled findings present evidence of a rather consistent pattern of the expected adverse effects for only one of the five parasites, *Ascaris.* The pattern for schistosomiasis also shows a sizable excess of the expected adverse effects, but the difference is not quite significant statistically. These results do suggest that there are some adverse effects of schistosomiasis and of *Ascaris* infection,[18] in addition to the earlier findings of significantly negative labor-productivity effects of the *Strongyloides* infection on women workers. When the pooled findings are combined with the findings reported earlier, that statistically significant effects were generally *not* found in the individual tests for schistosomiasis or for the other parasitic diseases, we are led to conclude that our varied

18. Additional examinations of the significance levels of disease coefficients showed that the average significance level of the coefficients with the *expected* sign, while not meeting the .10 level, was nonetheless greater than the average significance level of the coefficients having unexpected signs. The finding adds a bit more strength to the view that there probably are some adverse effects of schistosomiasis and the disease caused by *Ascaris.*

statistical efforts provide mild evidence of weak effects of schistosomiasis and two of the parasites—*Ascaris* and, to some extent, *Strongyloides*. Finally, the pooled findings reinforce the view that the five parasitic diseases, taken as a group, do bring adverse overall effects, particularly on labor productivity.

6

INTERPRETING
THE FINDINGS

This study has focused on the economic and social impact of schisto-somiasis and other parasitic infections in St. Lucia. Our findings are that, on the whole, infection by schistosomiasis and also by any of the other parasitic diseases studied appears to cause few statistically significant adverse effects on these variables. If it is true that parasites debilitate the body and thereby affect physical and mental performance, we would expect to find substantial effects. We have noted earlier, how-ever, that severe physiological effects of schistosomiasis or other parasitic diseases are believed to be a consequence not of all infections but of only the "relatively intensive" infections. Thus, it is possible that infection intensities found in St. Lucia are rarely if ever severe enough to bring about notable effects on behavior and performance. We shall return to this explanation later, as we consider in this chapter a number of answers to the question of why so little of the expected adverse effects appeared.

One possible reason for not finding large effects is simply errors in measurement; our data on parasite prevalence, labor productivity, school performance, birth and death rate, and so on may have been too imprecise for gauging the consequences of these parasites. This seems unlikely, however, given the considerable number of independent bodies of data utilized, the variety of population groups studied, and the alternative measures of effects that were considered.

More plausible is the possibility of serious model misspecification—

involving either the omission of relevant independent variables or an erroneous specification of the ways by which the independent variables affect the dependent variables (that is, the functional form). It is true that our models were able to explain only a small percentage of the observed variation in the various dependent variables.

Bear in mind that our complete view (hypothesis) was that structural relationships of two sorts exist: (1) between parasitic infections and the occurrence of physical and mental debility; and (2) between physical/ mental debility and the occurrence of adverse behavioral effects. In fact, we did not attempt to estimate these two sets of relationships separately, but rather we estimated reduced-form equations relating the presence of parasitic infections to the occurrence of adverse behavioral effects. Thus we cannot tell whether the limited behavioral effects that we found result from the lack of debilitation or from the absence of an effect of debilitation on performance, or both.

Another problem with our models as estimated is that they took into explicit account only some of the adverse effects which the diseases might bring about. Indeed, we did not set out to test for "all" effects, but only for certain effects that were likely to have "important" economic consequences. Yet it is possible that the failure to take other effects into account had an influence on our findings regarding the effects that we were testing for.

For example, although weekly money incomes were apparently not affected by the presence of any of the parasites, the composition of consumer expenditures and the saving-consumption ratio might be altered. If it is true, for example, that parasites reduce the proportion of nutrients from any given food intake that becomes available to the human body, then persons having parasites may devote a larger share of any given budget to food, in order to sustain their level of physiological and productive capability. Our initial research strategy included an investigation of budgetary behavior, but difficulties in obtaining useful data led us to drop these plans. It would be desirable in future work to test for the effects of diseases on saving and expenditure behavior, since the macroeconomic effects could be important.

This discussion has at least two noteworthy implications: one is that the parasites may have produced some consequences, even if not in the forms that were studied. The other is that if we had estimated a complete model in which these other consequences were considered and in which their possible feed-back effects on our "economic" variables were also considered, we might have arrived at a different set of conclusions regarding the effects of the parasites on the economic variables. More about this below.

The models we estimated were not able to control for all factors other than the parasitic diseases that affect, directly or indirectly, labor productivity, birth and death rates, or schoolchildren's academic performance, and that might vary systematically with these variables. In addition, although we did consider alternative forms of the equations that were estimated—in particular, the possibilities of interaction effects among diseases—the true forms of the relationships between the independent and dependent variables may be distinctly nonlinear or otherwise different from the forms actually estimated, and this is another source of potential model-misspecification error. Whether the appropriate explanation is omitted variables, incorrect functional form, or measurement errors, the fact remains that—as the low R^2 values of our estimates show—we are far indeed from being able to explain all of the variance in fertility, mortality, productivity, and school performance that our data disclosed.

The model-misspecification possibility has another dimension. Whereas our reduced-form equations, as estimated, implied that causation ran from the "independent" variables to the "dependent" variables, we have already questioned the validity of this assumption. Causation may run in both directions. For example, not only might it be true that children who are debilitated with schistosomiasis are absent from school more (or possibly less), but children who, for other reasons, are absent a great deal may be more likely to contract schistosomiasis as they play or work in infected streams rather than sit in the classroom. Similarly, workers with schistosomiasis or other parasites may be more likely to seek certain types of (non-physically-demanding) work, but it may also be true that workers who perform certain types of work are more likely to contract schistosomiasis.[1]

The possibility of such interdependencies suggests development of simultaneous equation models with lagged variables so that it would be possible to determine whether the parasitic infection preceded or followed the decisions concerning work or schooling. But the resources and data available for our study precluded investigation of time-series models.

As a result, it remains possible that our findings—of few significant associations between presence of any of the parasites and various types of performance—actually mask more significant relationships. If, for example, those agricultural workers who were most energetic and ambitious to begin with elected to do types of work which increased their parasite-infection rate and thereby decreased their productivity, they might still be as productive as their less energetic and ambitious co-workers for whom parasitic infections were less common or less severe. In such a

---

1. For further discussion of the latter point see Appendix H.

case investigators would find—as, to some extent, we did—no significant differences between the (weekly) productivity levels of infected and non-infected workers. The fact that we could not control, however, for all sources of relevant variation in initial characteristics of the individuals studied means that we cannot rule out the possibilities just discussed. We attempted to account for such variation by controlling for age, sex, and level of educational attainment—the latter viewed as a proxy for motivation—but the degree of our success is conjectural. It does not seem likely, however, that systematic selection processes were so consistently at work as to hide the effects of the parasites on all of the groups of people and in all of the forms of impact that we considered.

Up to this point we have considered reasons why we might have *found* no significant effects of the parasites even if such effects were actually present. Now we turn to explanations of why—contrary to our initial hypothesis—the parasitic infections in St. Lucia or elsewhere might actually have little or no significant effect on birth and death rates, labor productivity of adults, and performance of schoolchildren.

It may be true that the *severity* of parasitic infections was low in St. Lucia, and that significant effects occur only beyond some threshold level of severity. We did test for such a nonlinear relationship between labor productivity and schistosomiasis severity—as measured by the egg count (number of eggs per gram of stool)—but while this disclosed little of significance, it could be that the range of severity observed in our data is simply too small. It is apparently true that egg counts are positively correlated with prevalence rates, suggesting that in regions having the highest prevalence the people are being re-infected repeatedly. And the evidence does indicate that both prevalence and "severity" of schistosomiasis are *currently* lower in St. Lucia than they have been found to be in at least some other parts of the world, as Table 6.1 indicates.

It may be noted in the table that egg counts increase more than proportionately with the prevalence rate. If the egg count is a satisfactory measure of severity—and there is some doubt about this—then it could be true that our findings of few significant effects of schistosomiasis are indeed correct for St. Lucia and even for areas of the world with the range of severity found in St. Lucia, though not necessarily for other ranges. Data of the type presented in Table 6.1 are available for only a handful of the many schistosomiasis-infected areas of the world. Dr. Peter Jordan, however, Director of the Rockefeller Foundation's Research and Control Department in St. Lucia, has told us that he regards St. Lucia not as a unique schistosomiasis area but as one that is representative of a number of areas of generally moderate severity. (We return to this point

Table 6.1. Correlation between Schistosomiasis Prevalence and Egg Load Level

Location	Prevalence (percentage of 5–9 year-old children having schistosomiasis)	Eggs per gram
Roseau Valley, St. Lucia	11	5
Riche Fond Valley, St. Lucia	33	55
Cul-de Sac Valley, St. Lucia	35	105
Gameleira ("Zone 1"), Brazil	37	110
Mwanza, Tanzania	61	202
Gameleira ("Zone 2"), Brazil	73	376
Gameleira ("Zone 3"), Brazil	95	590

Note: This information was supplied by Dr. Peter Jordan, Director, St. Lucia Research and Control Department. The St. Lucian data are for 1968, the Tanzanian data for 1961, and the Brazilian data for 1961. The source for the Brazilian data is [90]. The other data are Jordan's, unpublished.

in chapter 7.) The table simply highlights the point that there are also parts of the world in which severity is more than "moderate."

If there is a nonlinearity in the function relating egg count to various impacts, it could, of course, apply outside the range of our observations. This is speculation, but it does provide the basis for a reminder that one's research findings apply, at most, within the range of observed data; extrapolation outside that range is always hazardous.

The nonlinearity possibility is important because there is the view that the prevalence of schistosomiasis in St. Lucia is growing, and with it the severity [234]. Thus, just as more substantial effects of the disease may already be found in other areas of the world—although there is little solid evidence of such effects—so they may be expected in St. Lucia at a later date. Whether or not this is true, no such argument has been made to explain our findings as to the general absence of negative effects of the other parasites—*Ascaris, Trichuris*, hookworm, and *Strongyloides*. Hookworm, in particular, has been endemic to St. Lucia for decades.

There remain two types of explanations for our findings, explanations that are consistent with the view that our findings are correct: namely that schistosomiasis and the other parasitic diseases in St. Lucia are currently having little if any effect on the demographic or school-performance variables studied and only weak effects on labor productivity. The first explanation is in terms of physiological adjustments; the second in terms of socio-cultural adjustments.

The human physiological system appears to have excess, or stand-by, capacity in a number of forms. Some forms, involving duplicate organs such as lungs, function in well-known ways. Others may be less apparent or less well understood but no less important. Parasitologists at the World Health Organization have stated in personal interviews the belief that such stand-by capacity may come into operation when the body is attacked by parasites. Thus, whereas the parasites would weaken the body and affect performance *if* other things remained constant, the physiological system adjusts, compensating for and offsetting the effects of parasitic infections. Since the ability of the system to compensate is presumably limited, very severe infection may produce serious and measurable consequences. This would explain the nonlinear severity function discussed above. Because of the belief that the body is capable of adjusting to, and compensating for, parasitic infection, physicians in the World Health Organization Parasitology Unit were not greatly surprised by our findings that, on the whole, there was little measurable effect of schistosomiasis and other parasitic diseases in St. Lucia.

What we have just said is that it is possible to have parasites without being bothered or affected by them because of physiological compensation. The possibility of "having" a disease without being "bothered" by it raises the question of what other factors might determine whether one is bothered by a disease, and this leads to a consideration of socio-cultural factors that influence the way people respond to disease.

People in an advanced Western society may curtail work effort in response to a given illness, while in another society the response may be to work harder or longer. A disease might debilitate and reduce the victim's *potential* labor productivity or academic performance or fertility level without reducing the *actual* level of any of these. Disease may not be the binding constraint on these forms of activity; preference patterns may be such that a decrease in overall capacity leads not to a reduction in all measures of activity, but only in some—and not in those examined in the present study.[2]

This line of reasoning suggests the hypothesis that in less-developed societies, such as St. Lucia, cultural factors may be important in explaining the forms of responses to disease. The following discussion will be in terms of the influence of these cultural factors on the manner in which disease may affect the labor productivity of adults, but much of the discussion may also be applicable to other performance variables such as

---

2. This type of explanation, however, does not seem applicable to the death rate; it is difficult (though not impossible) to see how that rate could be affected by extra-physiological factors.

achievement in school. The point is that cultural factors can influence whether the debilitating effects of disease—granted their presence—manifest themselves in the forms that we were interested in, or in other forms.[3]

In regard specifically to plantation workers, one such cultural force might explain why "healthier" workers may be no more productive than less healthy workers. Agricultural wage labor continues to be associated with slavery in St. Lucia despite the abolition of slavery in 1834; St. Lucian politicians do not hesitate to argue that only those workers who refuse to conform to the *béché* (white man's) method of oppression can be truly free. Indeed, knowledgeable observers have reported that many people in the West Indies would rather be idle than work as field hands in agriculture [188, p. 38]. The view of agricultural work as a loathsome activity, combined with the ease of subsistence in a warm climate where breadfruit, bananas, and coconuts are easily picked from estate lands without detection, contributes to a generally slow pace of economic activity [169, p. A-5].

Poverty and cultural life-style may thus be at least partly responsible for St. Lucians' having little incentive to work harder or longer even if physically capable of doing so. At this time we cannot reject, nor can we accept, the hypothesis that debilitation of spirit, not of body, is the binding constraint on the levels of social and economic activity in St. Lucia. Our findings in chapter 5 and appendices B, C, and D *may* be explainable at least partly by these socio-cultural influences. They may prevent parasitic infections from affecting *actual* productive performance, even when the infections do debilitate and even if their effects on potential performance are real and important. A question remains, however, regarding whether such "debilitation of spirit" is not itself dependent on individuals' objective opportunities and, hence, on their states of health.

In short, to know that some individuals are infected or even weakened by disease may not be sufficient to predict their productivity or academic performance compared with healthy people, because poor health is but one of the forces constraining behavior. In a society where cultivating extended family ties, assuaging the wrath of evil spirits, or enjoying increased leisure is deemed more important than augmenting money income or academic performance, the performance effects of parasitic diseases may be insignificant: not because the parasites are physiologically unimportant, but because the key to increased achievement-motivation lies in altering traditional beliefs and behavior patterns. Under these

---

3. The remainder of this section is drawn in part from an unpublished manuscript by Erwin H. Epstein [196].

circumstances, poor health might have substantial consequences indeed, but not in the forms of the performance variables that we studied.

These possibilities do indeed exist. Nevertheless, since we do find, in St. Lucia and in less-developed countries generally, that people do respond to economic incentives,[4] we are inclined to the view that socio-cultural factors are no more than partial explanations for our quantitative findings of weak effects of infection with schistosomiasis or the other individual parasites.

To summarize, there are a number of possible explanations for our findings of the little effect parasitic infections seem to have in St. Lucia:

1. Effects may have occurred but were not detected.
   a. The data may be weak.
   b. The model that was estimated may be incomplete or incorrectly specified, relevant variables having been omitted or the form of the relationships between the variables having been wrongly stated. The diseases may have caused debilitation, but because of the intervention of socio-cultural variables or for other reasons, the effects of diseases, while real, occurred in forms other than those studied.
2. There may actually have been no substantial effects on our three sets of performance variables.
   a. Adjustment of the human physiological system may have compensated for and offset the effects of the parasites.
   b. There may have been no observed effects of the parasitic infections in St. Lucia because the infections are not sufficiently severe, a situation that may be different in the future or may be different elsewhere in the world even now.

At present we cannot be certain which explanation is correct. Indeed, a number may be correct, and the same explanation need not be valid with respect to each of the relationships between a disease and a performance variable. Given the sizable number of relationships we considered and the variety of bodies of data examined, however, and the relative consistency of our negative findings, together with the fact that there were some positive findings (that the presence of the *Strongyloides* parasite was associated with lower fertility among women and lower labor productivity of women at work, and that schistosomiasis infection appears

---

4. The form and direction of the response, however, can vary. For one piece of evidence regarding the labor-supply response by one group in St. Lucia to an increase in the piece-work wage, see Appendix G.

to reduce male labor productivity per day), suggest to us that measurement errors are probably not the principal explanation. We lean to the view that severe effects of the parasites studied either have not occurred because physiological compensations have taken place, or, if they have occurred, have taken forms other than those we examined in our research. These judgments, however, remain hypotheses that require further testing. Similarly, the questions of whether schistosomiasis and the other parasitic diseases have larger impacts in other geographic areas (where either the *S. mansoni* or another schistosome species is found), or will have larger impacts later on, remain open.

It would be appropriate to end this chapter with our own best assessment of the importance of the factors discussed above. In our judgment, the quality, the quantity, and the variety of our data were quite satisfactory, on the whole. The possibility of model-misspecification always exists, but given the consistency of our independent results, we have some confidence that this is not at the root of our findings. In addition, our models—developed separately by each of several researchers—examined a number of alternative functional forms for the models but found no evidence that the general lack of disease-impact was due to nonlinearities; this leads us to believe that our findings are probably not attributable to incorrect identification of functional form. We conclude that the evidence is rather strong that schistosomiasis and the other parasitic diseases studied in St. Lucia are actually having only quite modest effects in any of the three broad areas we have investigated.

7

CONCLUDING
THOUGHTS

S chistosomiasis and the four other parasitic diseases studied here infect
  hundreds of millions of people—primarily in the developing parts of
the subtropical world. What effects are these diseases bringing? Are they
a major cause of low income and slow economic development in these
regions?

What Have We Found?

While our various bodies of data show little connection between the
presence of any of these parasites and either birth or death rates, achievement of children in school, or labor productivity of adults, our analysis
does show evidence of some adverse effect of schistosomal infection on
labor productivity. We do not argue that these parasites have no other
consequences—they may affect the quantity and quality of leisure time
and relationships within the household, for example—but we do conclude
that economic development is not being retarded importantly by their
presence.

It would be less than cautious to generalize to the entire world the
findings from a study of the impact of any disease in one area. Additional
case studies should be undertaken, particularly in areas of high prevalence
rates and high infection intensities, where there is prior reason to expect
substantial physiological effects of parasites. For now, it may be appro-

priate to note that the hundreds of millions of persons who are believed to be infected with some form of schistosomiasis include an unknown, but possibly quite large proportion whose infection levels are "moderate," as is the case in St. Lucia. As Table 7.1 indicates, many other areas have been found to have prevalence rates for schistosomiasis comparable to those found in St. Lucia. Ideally we would like to have information on both prevalence rates and some measure of intensity levels of schistosomiasis in various areas. Intensity measures, whether by egg counts or something else, however, are generally not available. Thus, in Table 7.1 we present a summary of schistosomiasis prevalence rates only, from recently published surveys, for St. Lucia and a number of other areas. It should be understood that the various studies summarized in the table apply to small communities, not to entire countries, and that the studies are not strictly comparable. The table does indicate, however, that the prevalence rates found in the St. Lucian studies are not at the low extreme of prevalence rates found elsewhere.

Whether the effects on economic development of the species of schistoso-

Table 7.1. Recent World-Wide Surveys of Prevalence Rates for Schistosomiasis (*S. mansoni*): Summary

Location	Prevalence
Sao Paulo, Brazil	1.1%
Ituri Forest, Congo	7.0
Ibadan, Nigeria	8.0
Gameleira, Brazil	8.8
Daiya, Nigeria	10.0
Nile Province, Uganda	13.0
Surinam	13.0
Yo, Nigeria	15.0
Ambositra, Madagascar	18.0
Soufriere, St. Lucia	*33.0*
Cul-de-Sac Valley, St. Lucia	*46.0*
Utinga, Brazil	
Males	47.0
Females	45.0
Nova Ouro, Brazil	53.0
Camboim, Brazil	63.0
Adwa, Ethiopia	
Males	65.0
Females	56.0
Rio Branco, Brazil	68.0
Harar, Ethiopia	71.0

Note: The studies cited above vary considerably in their sample size and in the ages of persons covered. See Appendix Table E.2 for details and source.

miasis found in St. Lucia, *Schistosoma mansoni,* can be generalized to the *S. haematobium* and *S. japonicum* varieties is another open question. There is some evidence that the *S. mansoni* species brings somewhat less severe physiological effects than the other forms of schistosomiasis [72, p. 527]. Thus, the effects on economic development of the other varieties could be greater than the effects of *S. mansoni.* In any event our findings for *S. mansoni* are notable because that species alone has been estimated to affect nearly thirty million people throughout not only the Caribbean but parts of Latin America and North and East Africa [72, pp. 517, 521].

A Final Note

With all the demands on resources to improve the lot of the world's poor, and with the limited resources available, particularly in the health area, choices must be made. Findings such as those reported here should, and do, enter the decision-making process as information (but not the only information) relevant to the question of how much resources are to be allocated among competing programs of disease prevention, control, and treatment. When the World Health Organization, for example, considers the desirability of launching an antidisease campaign in some poor area of the world, it must frequently turn for financing to the World Bank or other international lending institutions, which, in turn, demand information as to the "benefits" and "costs" of alternative programs, whether involving diseases, schools, roads, power, or some other developmental uses.

Quantitative findings from studies such as ours can be useful parts of the decision-making process, though judgments concerning the importance of unmeasured effects of disease should, and do, also enter. Empirical findings about schistosomiasis and other parasitic diseases constitute, however, only one form of output of this study. A second, we believe, was our partial success in pushing beyond the casual observations that characterize so many of the earlier estimates of the effects of disease in developing economies. Our determination to quantify as many "relevant" variables as possible led us to design a research strategy that involved gathering data on variables, such as achievement in school, that are often thought of as "noneconomic."

We believe that the approach employed in this study is useful as a prototype for other studies of disease effects. Yet study of the economic impact of disease is still in its infancy. It is possible to do rigorous quantitative work in this area. But, as this study has shown, the energies and talents of economists need to be combined with those of medical personnel and a larger social perspective to understand how man adjusts to disease.

APPENDICES

REFERENCES

INDEX

Appendix A

SURVEY INSTRUMENTS

The household survey, the Geest worker survey, and the Dimensions, Ltd., survey were all orally administered in St. Lucian patois by trained, bilingual (English and patois-speaking) St. Lucian interviewers. One interviewer conducted the household survey in the Cul-de-Sac Valley and another conducted the survey in the Roseau Valley. The Geest worker and Dimensions, Ltd., surveys were also each conducted by one interviewer. The school health survey was administered in the questionnaire form included in this appendix, with answers written on the forms by the pupils following instructions from a bilingual St. Lucian.

Household Survey (Revised Instructions)

1. Identification number

2. What is your name?

3. What is your age?
   (Age at last birthdate, e.g., $\frac{1}{12}$ year, $\frac{2}{12}$ year, ... ,
   $1\frac{1}{12}$, 1 year, 2 years, etc.)

5. What is your highest level of educational attainment?
   (For those still in school, the current level (e.g., standard) of educational attainment; for those out of school, the highest level

of educational attainment *completed* (by examination or some other plausible criterion). Use the same classifications found in the St. Lucia census: Kindergarten (K), Standard 1 (1), Standard 2 (2), ... , Secondary 1st year (8), Secondary 2nd year (9), . . . , University (U). The abbreviations in parentheses can be used to indicate the level of education).

7–8. How many children have you given birth to during the past 24 months?
(We desire the total number of *live* births *and* still births for each woman in the house. Indicate live births and still births separately. All births should be counted whether or not a birth certificate was issued or the child was baptized.)

9. Did you work for Geest Estates?
(This question should be asked of all members of the household who could have worked for Geest, whether full-time or part-time. The responses fall into three categories: Yes, Cul-de-Sac = C; Yes, Roseau = R; No = N.)

10. Other than employment on the Geest Estates, what work do you do?

11. What is your "work name"?
(This question is to be answered for those members of the household who work for Geest if their "work name" is different from either of those entered in cols. (1) or (2).)

12–14. During the last two years, did any member of your household leave for a period exceeding one month? If yes, complete cols. (12)–(14).

12. Where did this person migrate?
(Indicate specific geographic area, e.g., Cul-de-Sac, Roseau, Castries area, Dennery, Barbados, Miami, etc.)

13. How long was this person gone?
(Length of migration, to nearest month, e.g., 1 month, 2 months, etc.)

14. What was this person's specific job where he migrated?
(For example, cane cutter, banana boat loader for Geest, taxi driver, street cleaner.)

15. Did any member of your household leave during the past two years who does not plan to rejoin the household? If yes, indicate

the number using each of three destinations: Outside St. Lucia, Castries area, other.

16–18.   Did any member of your household die in the last 24 months? If yes, give name on death certificate, age, and sex of deceased.

School Health Survey Questionnaire

This is not an examination. The questions that follow do not have right or wrong answers. Your answers to the questions will not in any way affect your grades. They will not even be seen by your teacher. No one will know how you have answered the questions because you will not put your name on this sheet.

We are asking these questions in order to find out what children in your school think about many things that affect them. You and all the children in the class must answer carefully all of the questions. This is the only way we can know something about children in school.

Number _____

PART I

Place an "X" in the space which best describes you. Where you are not asked to place an X, answer the question as fully as you can.

1)   What are you? Place an "X" in the correct space.
_____a) boy
_____b) girl

2a)   Have you ever lived outside of St. Lucia?
_____a) yes   Where else? _____.
_____b) no

2b)   Have you ever lived outside of the area or district you presently live in?
_____a) yes   Where else? _____.
_____b) no

3)   What was the highest level of school that your father attended? Place an "X" in the correct space.
_____a) he never attended school
_____b) Infant (Stage I–Stage III)
_____c) Junior (Standard I–Standard IV)
_____d) Senior (Standard V–Standard VI)
_____e) Secondary (Form I–Form VI)

4) What was the highest level of school that your mother attended? Place an "X" in the correct space.

_____a) she never attended school
_____b) Infant (Stage I–Stage III)
_____c) Junior (Standard I–Standard IV)
_____d) Senior (Standard V–Standard VI)
_____e) Secondary (Form I–Form VI)

5a) What work does your father do? (Explain as fully as you can what he does, including for whom he works.) _____

_____

If your father is dead, what did he do? _____

_____

5b) What work does your mother do? _____

_____

Part II

Answer each question as completely as you can. Where the questions have alternative answers, choose the one that best answers the question for you.

1) Where does your family get water to drink?
_____a) from a stream.
_____b) from an irrigation canal.
_____c) from a pipe (tap).
_____d) from a water barrel.
_____e) from a well.

2) Where does your family bathe or get water in which to bathe?
_____a) from the sea.
_____b) from a stream.
_____c) from an irrigation canal.
_____d) from a pipe (tap).
_____e) from a water barrel.
_____f) from a well.

3) Where does your family get water in which to wash clothes?
_____a) from the sea.
_____b) from a stream.
_____c) from an irrigation canal.
_____d) from a pipe (tap).
_____e) from a water barrel.
_____f) from a well.

4a) Do you use a latrine?

    _____a) yes

    _____b) no

4b) Explain your reason for using or not using a latrine. _____

_____

5a) Is there a latrine in or near your home?

    _____a) yes

    _____b) no

5b) If there is a latrine in or near your home, about how long ago was it put there?

    _____a) more than six years ago.

    _____b) between three and six years ago.

    _____c) between one and three years ago.

    _____d) less than one year ago.

6a) Is water ever boiled in your home?

    _____a) yes

    _____b) no

6b) Explain the most important reason why water is or is not boiled in your home. _____

_____

7a) Are there any members of your family living in your home who have been very sick within the last two years, explain what is or was wrong with each of them. _____

_____

7b) Are there any members of your family living in your home who have been very sick within the last two years?

    _____a) yes

    _____b) no

PART III

Answer each question as completely as you can. Where the questions have alternative answers, choose the one that best answers the question for you.

1a) Which one of the following do you think is the best for drinking?

    _____a) water from a stream.

    _____b) water from an irrigation canal.

    _____c) water from a pipe (tap).

    _____d) rainwater from a barrel.

    _____e) water from a well.

1b)   Explain the most important reason for your answer. _____

_____

2a)   What kind of water do you think is the best for bathing?
_____a) water from the sea.
_____b) water from a stream.
_____c) water from an irrigation canal.
_____d) water from a pipe (tap).
_____e) rainwater in a barrel.
_____f) water from a well.

2b)   Explain the most important reason for your answer. _____

_____

3a)   Which kind of water do you think is the best for washing clothes?
_____a) water from the sea.
_____b) water from a stream.
_____c) water from an irrigation canal.
_____d) water from a pipe (tap).
_____e) rainwater from a barrel.
_____f) water from a well.

3b)   Explain the most important reason for your answer. _____

_____

4a)   Which one of the following places do you think is best to ease the
bowels?
_____a) stream.
_____b) canal.
_____c) latrine.
_____d) the field.

4b)   Explain the most important reason for your answer. _____

_____

Part IV

1)   What do you think usually causes people to become sick? _____

_____

2)   How do you know this? _____

_____

3)   If you were told this by somebody, who told you? _____

_____

Geest Worker Survey

1. What is your name?

2. What is your age?

3. What is your address? (Region of the valley in which household is located.)

4. What is your house number? (The number painted on the house by the Parasitological Survey team.)

5. Do you live in housing provided by Geest?

6. Do you live on Geest land?

7. What is the highest educational standard you have attained?

8. On average, how many hours per week do you work for Geest?

9. On average, how many hours per week do you work at all *other* jobs, including work on your own lands?

10. Other than your work at Geest, which is your most important work activity? Which is the second most important? Which is the third most important?

11. Do you grow your own bananas? If so, how many plants do you have?

12. During the last two years, did you leave Cul-de-Sac for a period of more than one month? If so, did you leave St. Lucia?

Dimensions, Ltd., Survey

1. What is your name?

2. What is your working team number?

3. What is your age?

4. What is the highest education standard you have attained?

5. What is the last school you attended?

6. What is your marital status, and if single, do you live alone or with your parents?

7. What is your religion?

8. How many children have you given birth to?
   (Indicate separately the number of live births and still births.)

9. Have you missed any work due to illness or other reasons?
   (Give approximate dates and the reason.)

10. How many dependents do you have?

11. What is your present address?

12. What have been your previous addresses? Give the approximate dates of when you lived there.

13. How often do you leave Castries, and where do you go?

Appendix B

TECHNICAL DISCUSSION OF THE NATALITY AND MORTALITY ANALYSIS

The sample selected for analysis of natality includes all women aged fifteen to forty-five for whom we have parasitological and educational information. The resulting sample size is 291 for Cul-de-Sac Valley and 241 for Roseau Valley. While this sample represents only 34 and 47 percent of the women aged fifteen to forty-five in Cul-de-Sac and Roseau, respectively, our statistical results are unbiased if we assume, as seems reasonable, that the households included in the analysis are generally representative of those in the two valleys. (For further discussion of the representativeness of these and our other samples, see Appendix F below.)

The birth rate, computed for each woman in the household, represents the number of children brought to term during the two-year interval prior to the household survey. The two-year period was selected in order to insure that the sample possessed a sufficient number of observations for statistical analysis. The parasitic-infection profile of the women in our sample is presented in Table B.1. This information is disaggregated by area of residence.

While the small sample size precludes analysis of all the possible parasite combinations, there are many combinations that occur with sufficient frequency to permit statistical investigation. In our analysis below we required at least five observations of a particular parasite combination for it to be included in the study.[1]

1. The statistical analysis utilizes maximum likelihood procedures. As D. J. Finney [11, p. 56] has noted, maximum likelihood procedures are inappropriate in the

Table B.1. Parasitic-Infection Profile of Roseau and Cul-de-Sac Valleys: Women, Ages 15–45

| | Parasite prevalence (alone or in combination with other parasites) | | | | | |
| | Cul-de-Sac | | Roseau | | Total | |
Parasite	Number	Percentage[a]	Number	Percentage[a]	Number	Percentage[a]
A	134	46.05	131	54.36	265	49.81
H	175	60.14	94	39.00	269	50.56
Sc	135	46.39	103	42.74	238	44.74
St	42	14.43	19	7.88	61	11.47
T	151	51.89	150	62.24	301	56.58

| | Prevalence of parasite combinations by number of parasites | | | | | |
| | Cul-de-Sac | | Roseau | | Total | |
Number of parasites	Number	Percentage[a]	Number	Percentage[a]	Number	Percentage[a]
0	15	5.15	20	8.29	35	6.57
1	58	19.93	51	21.16	109	20.48
2	106	36.42	80	33.19	186	34.96
3	84	28.86	75	31.11	159	29.88
4	25	8.59	14	5.80	39	7.33
5	3	1.03	1	.41	4	.75

| | Prevalence of parasite combinations by parasites | | | | | |
| | Cul-de-Sac | | Roseau | | Total | |
Parasite	Number	Percentage[a]	Number	Percentage[a]	Number	Percentage[a]
None	15	5.15	20	8.30	35	6.58
A	10	3.44	12	4.98	22	4.14
H	13	4.47	4	1.66	17	3.20
Sc	19	6.53	14	5.81	33	6.20
St	1	.34	1	.41	2	.38
T	15	5.15	20	8.30	35	6.58
A, H	15	5.15	3	1.24	18	3.38
A, Sc	12	4.12	12	4.98	24	4.51
A, St	0	0	1	.41	1	.19
A, T	12	4.12	24	9.96	36	6.77
H, Sc	20	6.87	9	3.73	29	5.45
H, St	6	2.06	2	.83	8	1.50
H, T	21	7.22	18	7.47	39	7.33
Sc, St	3	1.03	1	.41	4	.75
Sc, T	17	5.84	10	4.14	27	5.08
St, T	0	0	0	0	0	0
A, H, Sc	14	4.81	8	3.32	22	4.14
A, H, St	4	1.37	1	.41	5	.94
A, H, T	30	10.31	24	9.96	54	10.15
A, Sc, St	1	.34	1	.41	2	.38

Table B.1. (*Continued*)

Prevalence of parasite combinations by parasites

Parasite	Cul-de-Sac		Roseau		Total	
	Number	Percentage[a]	Number	Percentage[a]	Number	Percentage[a]
A, Sc, T	9	3.09	27	11.20	36	6.77
A, St, T	1	.34	3	1.24	4	.75
H, Sc, St	4	1.37	1	.41	5	.94
H, Sc, T	16	5.50	8	3.32	24	4.51
H, St, T	4	1.37	2	.83	6	1.13
Sc, St, T	1	.34	0	0	1	.19
A, H, Sc, St	3	1.03	1	.41	4	.75
A, H, Sc, T	11	3.78	9	3.73	20	3.76
A, H, St, T	9	3.09	3	1.24	12	2.26
A, Sc, St, T	0	0	1	.41	1	.19
H, Sc, St, T	2	.69	0	0	2	.38
A, H, Sc, St, T	3	1.03	1	.41	4	.75

Note: A = *Ascaris*, H = Hookworm, Sc = *Schistosoma*, St = *Strongyloides*, T = *Trichuris*.

[a] The percentage figures are based on the population surveyed in each of the individual valleys: Cul-de-Sac, 291; Roseau, 241.

We hypothesize (1) that schistosomiasis adversely affects the probability of giving birth, (2) that age is nonlinearly related to the birth rate, and (3) that higher educational attainment diminishes average family size. Before we undertake a statistical analysis of these hypotheses, however, we shall examine two problems that arise in translating these hypotheses into a form suitable for testing. First, the information on births applies to a two-year interval prior to the data recorded for parasite prevalence, education, and age. Ideally, we should utilize data on the level of each explanatory variable recorded at the *beginning* of the interval rather than at the end. The resulting measurement errors, however, may not be serious. Errors in the measurement of years of education completed are not likely to be important since the low level of educational attainment (a maximum of eight years) suggests that most of the women in the sample had completed their education prior to the two-year interval for which births were recorded. To a lesser degree, a similar observation applies to the data on parasite prevalence since the incidence rate (of *new* infection) tends to fall off dramatically by age twenty.

The measurement problem with respect to disease information is even more complicated if, as we noted above, the probability of contracting

small-sample case: ". . . a value less than five for the expected number in any class has often been taken as a warning that the chi-square distribution may give misleading results."

schistosomiasis is positively related to the duties of motherhood. Since these duties occur *after* the time of birth, and since our data on parasite infection also apply to the period after birth, then our data, as collected, are acceptable for testing the hypothesis that the probability of contracting schistosomiasis is higher in new mothers. Specifically, we wish to test the proposition that the presence of schistosomiasis for any particular woman is a function of the number of births, age, education, and region —that is, whether a woman does or does not have schistosomiasis is related to whether she gave birth to a child during the previous two years, her age (20, . . . , 45) her educational attainment (standards 0, . . . , 8), and the overall prevalence rate of schistosomiasis in her region of residence. The regional prevalence rates are for household groupings or "neighborhoods" within Cul-de-Sac Valley.[2] This variable is a proxy for the probability of a woman coming in contact with contaminated water in the immediate proximity of her home. In our tests we also allow for the possibility that the impact of age and education on the probability of contracting schistosomiasis varies according to the regional prevalence rate. We hypothesize that older persons in regions of high prevalence are less likely to be infected with schistosomiasis than are similar persons in low prevalence areas, since immunity to disease, taking time to develop, is directly related to the frequency of re-infection. We further hypothesize that the deterring effect of education on the probability of contracting schistosomiasis is greater the higher the regional prevalence rate. This is because health education, either in the school or at home, tends to emphasize the most important problems specific to the region.

Standard least-squares regression procedures are inadequate for this type of problem since the dependent variable is in binary form. We have thus used probit analysis, a statistical technique appropriate when the dependent variable is dichotomous [12, pp. 250–251]. Each observation is assumed to possess a "threshold" level, above which the dependent variable assumes a value of 1 and below which it assumes a value of 0. An index, I, is formed, which is a linear (in parameters) combination of the variables; I can be compared with the threshold level to determine whether the dependent variable assumes a value of 0 or 1. Maximum likelihood procedures are employed.[3]

2. These household groupings have been provided by Dr. Ronald Lees, a researcher formerly on the staff of the Rockefeller Foundation schistosomiasis research project (Research and Control Department) in St. Lucia.

3. A detailed discussion of probit analysis is found in [11] [22]. The statistic, $-2 \log \lambda =$ the likelihood ratio, possesses a chi-square distribution. It is assumed that the maximum likelihood estimates are asymptotically normal; thus, the standard normal distribution is used to assess the significance of the estimated parameters.

Equation (1) presents the results of the statistical test with standard errors of estimate in parentheses beneath the regression coefficients:

(1) schistosomiasis = -3.02*** + .06 Births + .03 Age + .04 Education
     (.84)   (.19)   (.03)   (.16)
   + 8.68*** Region − .14*** Age · Region − 1.09 Education · Region
    (1.98)   (.05)   (.61)
   + .73 Education · Region$^{1/2}$.
    (.62)

*** = Significant coefficient at the .01 level.

The specific functional form of the interaction terms was selected on the basis of considerable statistical experimentation in which it was found that expression (1) obtained the highest value of the likelihood function. The results of the test fail, however, to support the hypothesis that the probability of contracting schistosomiasis is positively related to the birth rate. Thus, in our empirical analysis below we shall assume that causation runs from schistosomiasis to births. This must be a guarded conclusion, however. If, in fact, the values of the variables at the end of the two-year period are equal to those at the beginning of the period, then it might be argued that the above test was not sufficient to reject the hypothesis that the prevalence of schistosomiasis is positively affected by the birth rate. This qualification must be borne in mind when appraising our empirical findings.

The difference between our two birth-rate hypotheses (an interaction model and an additive model) can be seen by considering an example in which the probability of giving birth, B, is assumed to be related to two diseases, D_1 and D_2, where $D_1 = 1$ if the disease is present, and 0 if it is not; $D_2 = 1$ if the disease is present, and 0 if it is not; $D_1D_2 = 1$ if both D_1 and D_2 are present, and 0 if they are not; and e is an error term. The interaction (general) model would be written as follows:

(2) $B = a + b_1D_1 + b_2D_2 + b_3D_1D_2 + e$ (interaction).

In contrast, the additive model would take the form

(3) $B = a' + b_1'D_1 + b_2'D_2 + e'$ (additive).

Table B.2 presents the probit results of the interaction model. Considerable experimentation was undertaken to assess the best functional form for the age and education variables; a nonlinear formulation using squared terms, by an examination of the probit residuals, yields the most accurate representation of the relationships under consideration. Since the remaining variables are all dichotomous, functional form is not relevant. We did insist, however, that each term included possess at least five observations (see footnote 1 to this appendix). In the probits for Cul-de-Sac and Roseau valleys, fourteen and eighteen disease combinations were

Table B.2. Interaction Model Probit Results for Cul-de-Sac and Roseau Valleys, Births as Dependent Variable

| Variable | Cul-de-Sac (N = 291) | | Roseau (N = 241) | |
	Coefficient	Standard error	Coefficient	Standard error
Intercept	−12.45***	1.69	−8.41***	1.39
Age	.87***	.12	.58***	.09
Age squared	−.015***	.002	−.009***	.001
Education	.15	.14	.46***	.14
Education squared	−.024	.019	−.067***	.020
A	−.61	.49	.89*	.51
H	.35	.42	—	—
Sc	.89**	.42	.52	.44
T	.46	.47	−.17	.35
A, H	.62	.42	—	—
A, Sc	2.12***	.57	−.13	.42
A, T	−.80	.62	.16	.34
H, Sc	−.19	.40	.53	.51
H, St	−3.32	3.21	—	—
H, T	.66	.39	.35	.38
Sc, T	−.59	.47	.12	.48
A, H, Sc	.84*	.46	−.26	.50
A, H, T	.54	.35	.71*	.37
A, Sc, T	.64	.59	.97***	.36
H, Sc, T	.34	.45	−.95	.61
H, Sc, St	−2.23	3.43	—	—
A, H, Sc, T	−.025	.90	−2.46	6.11
A, H, St, T	−.043	.52	—	—

Note: A = *Ascaris*, H = Hookworm, Sc = *Schistosoma*, St = *Strongyloides*, T = *Trichuris*. Each variable possessed at least five observations (dashes indicate fewer than five observations). See footnote 3 to this appendix for a discussion of the significance tests. $-2 \log \lambda$ yields 78.64 and 45.98 for Cul-de-Sac and Roseau, respectively.
  * Significant coefficient at the .10 level (two-tailed test).
  ** Significant coefficient at the .05 level (two-tailed test).
  *** Significant coefficient at the .01 level (two-tailed test).

omitted, respectively. When variables are omitted from the analysis, an issue arises as to the interpretation of the statistical results. In particular, while individual parasite combinations with less than five observations may not be reliably estimated, or even statistically significant, their *joint* impact may in fact exert a significant influence on births. If this were the case, the interpretation of each of the remaining parasite combinations in the probit would be relative to the *average* influence of the omitted variables. We have therefore tested the hypothesis that those variables omitted jointly influence the probability of giving birth. For each valley this hypothesis was rejected. Thus, the parasite combinations remaining in the probits can be interpreted as the impact of each variable on the probability of a woman giving birth during the two-year period under study.

In both valleys the nonlinear relationship between age and births is highly significant and accords with a priori expectations. While the estimated parameters for Cul-de-Sac and Roseau are quite different, both yield predictions showing the probability of births rising to around age thirty, and declining thereafter.[4]

The results showing the impact of education on births are more difficult to interpret. In Cul-de-Sac education does not exert a statistically significant impact on births, while in Roseau the impact is significant. In the latter case, the association of births and education is positive up to education level Standard 3, turning negative thereafter. The positive impact up to Standard 3 diminishes very rapidly, and the negative impact after this education level becomes increasingly powerful as the educational attainment of the mother rises.[5] A positive relationship between births and education at low education levels may be explained by the dominance of the income over the substitution effect in this range of the function. As education (and, we assume, income) levels rise, however, the opportunity costs of children also rise and the substitution effect becomes relatively more powerful.

The more restrictive, additive model relating births and health was discussed in chapter 5, and Table B.3 presents probit results for this model in which each parasite is entered individually and all interaction terms are omitted.

Table B.4 presents the five-year death record for each of the areas within the Cul-de-Sac and Roseau valleys.[6] The overall death rate of the 1968 population is implausibly low. However, the hypothesis to be tested is that the between-region variation is explained in part by the prevalence of schistosomiasis, after controlling for other factors influencing mortality. If the degree of understatement of deaths is not related to these other factors employed in the analysis of death rates, then our resulting estimates are not biased by the underreporting of the mortality data.

The variables used to explain death rates are taken from the household surveys of the valleys. By overlaying the valley survey maps showing

4. The index in age reaches a maximum at age thirty for Cul-de-Sac and thirty-two for Roseau.

5. A "Standard" is an education level in the St. Lucian school system. The probit index in education alone for Standards 1–8 yields, respectively, .393, .652, .777, .768, .625, .348, −.063, −.608.

6. Even though death records were available for other rural and urban areas in St. Lucia, the unavailability of information on parasite prevalence precluded an expansion of the sample.

Table B.3. Additive Model Probit Results for Cul-de-Sac and Roseau Valleys, Births as Dependent Variable

Variable	Cul-de-Sac (N = 291)		Roseau (N = 241)	
	Coefficient	Standard error	Coefficient	Standard error
Intercept	−10.0753***	1.2815	−7.4232***	1.1761
Age	0.7092***	0.0871	0.5027***	0.0809
Age squared	−0.0120***	0.0015	−0.0084***	0.0014
Education	0.2185	0.1522	0.5990***	0.1744
Education squared	−0.0264	0.0166	−0.0703***	0.0196
Ascaris	0.4034**	0.1732	0.2049	0.1844
Hookworm	0.0220	0.1823	−0.0826	0.1913
Schistosoma	0.0123	0.1811	−0.2086	0.1912
Strongyloides	−1.0716***	0.2796	−1.1202***	0.3800
Trichuris	−0.2511	0.1713	−0.1045	0.1930

Note: See footnote 3 to this appendix for a discussion of the significance test. −2 log λ yields 80.6 for Cul-de-Sac and 49.7 for Roseau.

** Significant coefficient at the .05 level (two-tailed test).

*** Significant coefficient at the .01 level (two-tailed test).

house numbers onto maps delineating areas by place names (corresponding to the death records), house-number groupings corresponding to the death-record place names were obtained. Using these groupings, data have been assembled for each neighborhood on its total population size, average age, sex ratio, and on the prevalence rate of each of the parasites under investigation.

The basic model relating death rates (noninfant) to schistosomiasis hypothesizes

$$(4) \quad (D/N) = f(\bar{A}, M/N, Sc^+/N, H^+N, A^+/N, T^+/N, St^+/N),$$

where D = deaths of persons greater than five years of age,
N = total population greater than five years of age,
$\bar{A}$ = mean age of population N,
M = males more than five years old,
Sc^+ = population in N showing *Schistosoma* positive,
H^+ = population in N showing hookworm positive,
A^+ = population in N showing *Ascaris* positive,
T^+ = population in N showing *Trichuris* positive,
St^+ = population in N showing *Strongyloides* positive.[7]

7. Studies by Victor R. Fuchs [35] and Richard Auster, Irving Leveson, and Deborah Sarachek [24] show that income, education, and availability of medical care help explain variations in death rates across states of the United States. Unfortunately, data on income are not available in our sample. Furthermore, across the rural St. Lucian regions considered in this study, there is little variation in either average education level or in the availability of medical facilities.

Table B.4. Deaths and Population by Area, Cul-de-Sac and Roseau Valleys, 1964–1968

Area	Deaths	Population (1967)	Deaths/100
Cul-de-Sac Valley			
Bar Denis	13	159	8.2
Beausejour; St. Joseph	5	249	2.1
Bexon	21	481	4.4
Ciceron	26	301	8.6
Goodlands	8	297	2.7
Joliment (Toorat)	5	101	5.0
La Bayse	14	744	1.9
Marc	20	344	5.8
Morne-Fortune	6	176	3.4
Odsan	10	236	2.4
Ti Colon	11	270	4.1
Roseau Valley			
Boisden	6	188	3.2
Jacmel	10	199	5.0
Jn. Baptiste	9	113	7.9
Marigot-de-Roseau	16	241	6.6
Millet	29	501	5.8
Morne D'Or	7	136	5.1

Note: Areas were omitted where there were fewer than five observations. Furthermore, La Croix Maingot, the location of the health center, was omitted. The total population estimates were obtained from the household survey.

The analysis was limited to the population greater than five years of age for two reasons. First, the prevalence of schistosomiasis in young children is almost negligible. Second, and more important, the overall death rate for infants and young children is very high, resulting in a nonlinear relationship between deaths and age which is very difficult to capture by a single statistic. By increasing the number of variables to capture this nonlinearity, we would simultaneously diminish the degrees of freedom, already a constraining factor given the small number of observations.

Expression (4), which relates death rates to various explanatory variables, possesses a basic specification error which should be recognized. While the death rate and the average age of persons in a region are postulated to be positively related, it is clear that as the variables are defined, the end-of-period mean age was influenced by the death rate in the previous years. Thus, high death rates among older persons may be associated with areas recording a low mean age. There seems to be no way of appraising the severity of this problem.[8]

A priori we would hypothesize that the impact on deaths of each explanatory variable—age, sex ratio, and disease prevalence—increases with its absolute level. The nonlinear relationship for age is well documented in the standard life-tables. However, since our age statistic represents an area's mean age, a lack of variation in this variable may make the issue of functional form unimportant; furthermore, for the same reason, the likelihood of the variable entering as a significant determinant of deaths is not great. Similarly, nonlinearities may be expected with respect to the disease variables. That is, if one postulates that the area's prevalence level is a rough proxy for the *intensity* of the disease, then the death rate should increase more than proportionately as the area's disease prevalence rate rises. This hypothesis can be captured by a logarithmic-linear functional form in which the estimated coefficient is greater than unity. The results of this regression calculation are presented in the right side of Table B.5, while the left side shows estimates of a linear formulation.

Table B.5. Regression Results in Cul-de-Sac and Roseau Valleys: Deaths as Dependent Variable

Independent variable	Linear formulation		Logarithmic-linear formulation	
	b_1 (1)	t-value (2)	b_1 (3)	t-value (4)
Intercept	−10.67	−1.00	−8.33	−1.30
Mean age, $\bar{A}$	.05	.13	.20	.05
Percentage male	.20	1.57	4.32	1.63
Percentage *Schistosoma*[+]	−.05	−.85	−.10	−.33
Percentage hookworm[+]	.08	1.11	1.03	1.26
Percentage *Ascaris*[+]	.00	.00	.17	.30
Percentage *Trichuris*[+]	−.03	−.60	−.55	−.86
Percentage *Strongyloides*[+]	−.11	−.65	−.20	.61
R^2	.41		.46	
Degrees of freedom	8		8	

Note: All variables apply to the population aged five years and older. None of the coefficients in the table are significant at the .10 level (two-tailed test).

8. As an experiment we constructed an instrumental variable in which the instrument, I_a, was a function of the other arguments in (4). The results are similar to those in Table B.5; moreover the basic conclusions of this section are not altered or qualified by these alternative estimates. Similar specification problems exist for each of the other variables in the analysis to the extent that these variables in fact have an impact on mortality.

While our findings (in Table B.5) are not statistically significant, two guarded observations may be in order. First, it is somewhat disconcerting to note that the coefficients of many of the parasite variables had negative signs, a result which we consider theoretically unacceptable. Second, hookworm appears to be the most serious candidate for possessing an impact on mortality. Since the lack of significance of this variable—the only parasite measure to possess a "correct" sign—may be due to a degree-of-freedom problem, an experiment was performed in which the log (D/N) was regressed on (M/N) and (H$^+$/N). This experiment can be justified by assuming that the impact of each of the omitted parasite variables on the death rate is zero. The results revealed that the significance level on the hookworm variable increased slightly, but still not to a statistically significant level.

Appendix C

TECHNICAL DISCUSSION OF THE ACADEMIC ACHIEVEMENT OF SCHOOL-CHILDREN ANALYSIS

Table C.1 shows the prevalence of schistosomiasis in the Cul-de-Sac Valley by age group and indicates the high prevalence rate among school-age children. The question in which we are interested is the effect on school-children—and, in particular, on their academic achievement—of infection with schistosomiasis and other parasitic diseases. The independent variables used for the study of students' academic performance are listed in Table C.2. Rather than distinguishing simply between urban and rural areas, our residence categories (Castries, other urban, and rural) take account of the importance of Castries as the island's social and economic center; the socio-economic distinctiveness of that city is displayed, for example, by the fact that in Castries 88 percent of the male population aged fifteen years and over went further in school than Standard 5, and 13 percent of the male working population held nonmanual jobs, in contrast to only 26 percent who finished higher in school than Standard 5 and eight percent who filled nonmanual positions in the total male population (including Castries) [187, vol. 2, pp. 8B–1, 18–1, and 19–1]. Our family-background variables serve as proxies for motivation and knowledge generated in the home, factors that must be considered if we are to explain variation in school performance.

Scores on the Nelson Reading Test for Grades 3–9 were used as the index of scholastic performance—the dependent variable [216]. That test contains 175 items: 100 items to measure vocabulary and 75 items

Table C.1. Prevalence of Schistosomiasis by Age Group in Cul-de-Sac Valley, 1967

Age (years)	Persons tested	Percentage with schistosomiasis
under 1	71	1.4
1	109	4.6
2	119	8.4
3	127	25.2
4	107	36.4
5	128	25.8
6	103	38.8
7	100	36.0
8	115	47.8
9	80	50.0
10–14	397	57.7
15–19	252	58.3
20–24	146	46.6
25–29	139	38.8
30–34	154	31.2
35–39	145	34.5
40–44	130	31.5
45–49	119	32.8
50–54	86	30.2
55–59	70	32.9
60–64	63	39.7
65–69	47	27.7
70–74	28	21.4
75–79	9	33.3
80–84	13	46.2
85–89	6	16.7

Source: [95] (data compiled from original survey forms).

to measure reading comprehension. Each reading-comprehension paragraph is followed by three questions, one pertaining to its general significance, one to knowledge of detailed information contained therein, and one aimed at assessing ability to predict probable outcomes from the situation depicted in the paragraph.

Table C.2 shows the mean and standard deviation of the dependent variable (scholastic performance) and each of the independent variables for which data were obtained in the aggregate sample.[1] The mean and

1. It was decided not to take account of the time and day of the week the examination was given and the length of time the students spent on the examination; these variables were thought to be uncorrelated with the independent variables, and, hence, their omission should not bias the estimates of the coefficients of the independent variables.

Table C.2. Means and Standard Deviations of Variables Used in the Island-Wide Survey of Schoolchildren, St. Lucia, 1968, Aggregate Sample

Variable	Mean	Standard deviation
Scholastic performance		
(Nelson Reading Test scores)	50.570	23.520
Schistosoma		
(1 if present, 0 if not)	0.127	0.334
Hookworm		
(1 if present, 0 if not)	0.253	0.436
Ascaris		
(1 if present, 0 if not)	0.513	0.501
Trichuris		
(1 if present, 0 if not)	0.595	0.492
Strongyloides		
(1 if present, 0 if not)	0.044	0.206
Castries		
(1 if resident, 0 if not)	0.361	0.482
Other urban		
(1 if resident, 0 if not)	0.367	0.484
Rural		
(1 if resident, 0 if not)	0.272	0.446
Father's education		
(1 if father reached Standard		
5 or above,[a] 0 if not)	0.614	0.488
Father's occupation		
(1 if father has high-status		
occupation,[b] 0 if not)	0.158	0.366
Knowledge of germ theory		
(1 if germ theory *not* indicated		
as cause of disease, 0 if indicated)	0.475	0.501
Family's source of water for		
drinking		
(1 if hazardous, 0 if safe)	0.082	0.276
Family's source of water for		
bathing		
(1 if hazardous, 0 if safe)	0.146	0.354
Family's source of water for		
laundering		
(1 if hazardous, 0 if safe)	0.202	0.403

Note: N = 158.

 [a] Standard 5 represents the first grade in the "Senior" level classification, the most advanced of three general categories of primary schooling. Of the 158 pupils tested for parasites, information on father's education was not available for 27, the latter being eliminated as observations for the variable "Father's education." Education of head of household was used as a proxy for father's education when the father was absent and his education unknown.

 [b] Occupational classifications were derived from such considerations as professional standing, skill level, and ownership of property. Father's occupation was considered a less exact, though perhaps equally important, indicator of socio-economic status than father's education. Inasmuch as the great majority of St. Lucian men hold unskilled or otherwise menial jobs, it was difficult to make accurate distinctions in status among most of them. Hence, it was decided to place individuals with distinctively "better" jobs—representing 16 percent of the fathers—in the "high" category. Information on father's occupation was not available for 9 of the 158 pupils tested for parasites, the 9 being eliminated as observations for the variable "Father's occupation." As in the case of father's education, occupation of head of household was used as a proxy for father's occupation when the father was absent and his occupation unknown.

Table C.3a. Means and Standard Deviations of Variables Used in the Island-Wide Survey of Schoolchildren, St. Lucia, 1968, Showing Castries Schoolchildren

Variable	Mean	Standard deviation
Scholastic performance		
(Nelson Reading Test scores)	63.740	21.980
Schistosoma		
(1 if present, 0 if not)	0.158	0.368
Hookworm		
(1 if present, 0 if not)	0.228	0.423
Ascaris		
(1 if present, 0 if not)	0.421	0.498
Trichuris		
(1 if present, 0 if not)	0.561	0.501
Strongyloides		
(1 if present, 0 if not)	0.053	0.225
Father's education		
(1 if father reached standard		
5 or above,[a] 0 if not)	0.702	0.462
Father's occupation		
(1 if father has high-status		
occupation,[a] 0 if not)	0.175	0.384
Knowledge of germ theory		
(1 if germ theory *not* indicated		
in cause of disease, 0 if indicated)	0.614	0.491
Family's source of water for		
drinking		
(1 if hazardous, 0 if safe)	0.017	0.132
Family's source of water for		
bathing		
(1 if hazardous, 0 if safe)	0.000	0.000
Family's source of water for		
laundering		
(1 if hazardous, 0 if safe)	0.035	0.186

Note: N = 57.

[a] See footnotes to Table C.2.

standard deviation of each of these variables for pupils in Castries, pupils in other urban areas, and rural schoolchildren are shown in Tables C.3a, C.3b, and C.3c. Correlation matrices are given for the island-wide sample and each of the disaggregated samples in Tables C.4a, C.4b, C.4c, and C.4d.

As for the prevalence rate of schistosomiasis for the island as a whole, available reports are disturbingly inconsistent. Estimates based on surveys of the school population range from 16 percent [119, p. 1] to 35 percent

Table C.3b. Means and Standard Deviations of Variables Used in the Island-Wide Survey of Schoolchildren, St. Lucia, 1968, Showing Other Urban Schoolchildren

Variable	Mean	Standard deviation
Scholastic performance		
(Nelson Reading Test scores)	48.500	22.220
Schistosoma		
(1 if present, 0 if not)	0.069	0.256
Hookworm		
(1 if present, 0 if not)	0.224	0.421
Ascaris		
(1 if present, 0 if not)	0.638	0.485
Trichuris		
(1 if present, 0 if not)	0.690	0.467
Strongyloides		
(1 if present, 0 if not)	0.017	0.131
Father's education		
(1 if father reached standard		
5 or above,[a] 0 if not)	0.672	0.473
Father's occupation		
(1 if father has high-status		
occupation,[a] 0 if not)	0.121	0.329
Knowledge of germ theory		
(1 if germ theory *not* indicated		
in cause of disease,		
0 if indicated)	0.379	0.489
Family's source of water for		
drinking		
(1 if hazardous, 0 if safe)	0.017	0.131
Family's source of water for		
bathing		
(1 if hazardous, 0 if safe)	0.069	0.256
Family's source of water for		
laundering		
(1 if hazardous, 0 if safe)	0.121	0.329

Note: N = 58.

[a] See footnotes to Table C.2.

[98] to 59 percent.[2] Our sample of Standard 6 and Form 2 schoolchildren displays the lowest rate of all—13 percent—which is surprising, particularly in view of the fact that individuals in the age-group we surveyed are

2. The 59 percent prevalence rate is based on tests using intradermal antigen injections of pupils in seventeen schools outside of Castries [119, p. 9]. That this estimate is so much higher than the others might merely reflect a greater sensitivity to mild infection of skin testing as opposed to stool testing. Yet M. K. Panikkar's figure of 35 percent applied to both stool testing and skin testing [98].

Table C.3c. Means and Standard Deviations of Variables Used in the Island-Wide Survey of Schoolchildren, St. Lucia, 1968, Showing Rural Schoolchildren

Variable	Mean	Standard deviation
Scholastic performance		
(Nelson Reading Test scores)	35.910	17.070
Schistosoma		
(1 if present, 0 if not)	0.163	0.373
Hookworm		
(1 if present, 0 if not)	0.326	0.474
Ascaris		
(1 if present, 0 if not)	0.465	0.505
Trichuris		
(1 if present, 0 if not)	0.512	0.506
Strongyloides		
(1 if present, 0 if not)	0.070	0.258
Father's education		
(1 if father reached Standard		
5 or above,[a] 0 if not)	0.419	0.499
Father's occupation		
(1 if father has high-status		
occupation,[a] 0 if not)	0.186	0.394
Knowledge of germ theory		
(1 if germ theory *not* indicated		
cause of disease, 0 if indicated)	0.419	0.499
Family's source of water for		
drinking		
(1 if hazardous, 0 if safe)	0.256	0.441
Family's source of water for		
bathing		
(1 if hazardous, 0 if safe)	0.442	0.502
Family's source of water for		
laundering		
(1 if hazardous, 0 if safe)	0.535	0.505

Note: N = 43.

[a] See footnotes to Table C.2.

presumed to be those most likely to have the parasite. While the other surveys sampled more schoolchildren, they gave no indication of using sampling techniques appropriate to insuring representativeness and covered less than half as many schools as did ours.

To estimate the effect of schistosomiasis on test scores, we first fitted the following equation:

$$S = a + \sum_{i=1}^{5} B_i X_i,$$

Table C.4a. Correlation Matrix, Island-Wide Survey of Schoolchildren, St. Lucia, 1968, Showing Aggregate Sample

	Schistosoma	Hookworm	Ascaris	Trichuris	Strongyloides	Castries	Other urban	Rural	Father's education	Father's occupation	Knowledge of germ theory	Family's source of water for drinking	Family's source of water for bathing	Family's source of water for laundering
Scholastic performance	-.09	-.07	-.08	.01	.03	.42	-.07	-.38	.25	.21	-.14	-.17	-.16	-.29
Schistosoma		.04	.03	.12	-.08	.07	-.13	.07	-.01	-.11	.02	.16	.11	.14
Hookworm			.01	.21	.02	-.04	-.05	.10	.01	-.09	.06	.09	.05	-.08
Ascaris				.18	-.04	-.13	.10	-.06	-.12	-.20	-.14	-.03	-.03	.08
Trichuris					.05	-.05	.15	-.10	.03	-.10	.06	.01	-.02	-.03
Strongyloides						.03	-.10	.08	-.02	-.01	.10	-.05	-.00	-.03
Castries									.13	.03	.21	-.18	-.31	-.31
Other urban									.09	-.08	-.14	-.18	-.16	-.15
Rural									-.24	.05	-.07	.30	.51	.51
Father's education										.17	-.03	-.09	-.11	-.12
Father's occupation											-.00	-.00	.02	-.00
Knowledge of germ theory												-.05	-.05	-.04
Family's source of water for drinking													.46	.48
Family's source of water for bathing														.68

Note: N = 158.

Table C.4b. Correlation Matrix, Island-Wide Survey of Schoolchildren, St. Lucia, 1968, Showing Castries Schoolchildren

	Schistosoma	Hookworm	Ascaris	Trichuris	Strongyloides	Father's education	Father's occupation	Knowledge of germ theory	Family's source of water for drinking	Family's source of water for bathing	Family's source of water for laundering
Scholastic performance	-.11	-.16	-.06	-.05	-.08	-.08	.41	-.35	-.24	.00	-.20
Schistosoma		.11	.02	.29	-.10	.07	-.07	-.15	.31	.00	.44
Hookworm			.13	.14	-.13	-.01	-.25	.09	-.07	.00	.12
Ascaris				.40	-.20	-.14	-.30	-.05	-.11	.00	-.16
Trichuris					-.11	-.03	-.34	.24	.12	.00	.17
Strongyloides						-.02	.10	.19	-.03	.00	-.04
Father's education							.10	-.04	.09	.00	.12
Father's occupation								-.11	-.06	.00	-.09
Knowledge of germ theory									.11	.00	.15
Family's source of water for drinking										.00	.70
Family's source of water for bathing											.00

Note: N = 57.

Table C.4c. Correlation Matrix, Island-Wide Survey of Schoolchildren, St. Lucia, 1968, Showing Other Urban Schoolchildren

	Schistosoma	Hookworm	Ascaris	Trichuris	Strongyloides	Father's education	Father's occupation	Knowledge of germ theory	Family's source of water for drinking	Family's source of water for bathing	Family's source of water for laundering
Scholastic performance	−.07	−.05	−.14	−.08	.19	.38	.14	−.13	−.03	−.07	−.30
Schistosoma		.18	.20	.03	−.04	.04	−.10	.07	−.04	.19	.11
Hookworm			−.02	.36	−.07	−.06	.05	.18	−.07	−.15	−.20
Ascaris				.04	.10	−.22	−.16	−.30	.10	−.08	.17
Trichuris					.09	−.07	−.09	−.09	.09	.03	.02
Strongyloides						.09	−.05	−.10	−.02	−.04	−.05
Father's education							.26	−.14	−.19	−.10	−.19
Father's occupation								.14	−.05	−.10	−.14
Knowledge of germ theory									.17	.07	.15
Family's source of water for drinking										.49	.36
Family's source of water for bathing											.53

Note: N = 58.

122

Table C.4d. Correlation Matrix, Island-Wide Survey of Schoolchildren, St. Lucia, 1968, Showing Rural Schoolchildren

	Schistosoma	Hookworm	Ascaris	Trichuris	Strongyloides	Father's education	Father's occupation	Knowledge of germ theory	Family's source of water for drinking	Family's source of water for bathing	Family's source of water for laundering
Scholastic performance	−.17	.20	.06	.24	.14	.24	.12	−.33	.06	.29	.19
Schistosoma		−.17	−.03	.05	−.12	−.12	−.21	.14	.17	.11	.32
Hookworm			−.05	.18	.20	−.19	−.08	−.09	.16	.08	−.25
Ascaris				−.02	.11	−.03	−.09	.06	−.01	.01	.21
Trichuris					.27	.17	.23	.07	.04	.03	−.07
Strongyloides						−.05	−.13	.14	.05	−.06	−.11
Father's education							.20	.04	.04	.10	.13
Father's occupation								−.04	−.01	.06	.09
Knowledge of germ theory									−.17	−.09	−.15
Family's source of water for drinking										.34	.33
Family's source of water for bathing											.64

Note: N = 43.

123

where S stands for reading test score, a is a constant term, and the X_i (i = 1, 2, . . . , 5) are dummy variables that represent parasitic infections; a given variable equaled 1 if the parasite it represented was present. The B_i are the estimated coefficients. Table C.5 shows the results of ordinary least-squares linear regressions with the Nelson Reading Test score as the dependent variable. The regression results show that the presence or absence of parasitic infections—taken one at a time—is not significant in explaining achievement scores.

In addition to estimating the effects merely of parasitic infections, we fitted an equation that also included dummy variables for residence in Castries, residence in other urban areas, source of water for drinking,

Table C.5. Additive Model Regression Coefficients (and Standard Errors), Parasites and Background Data as Independent Variables and Reading Test Scores as Dependent Variable

Constant	Schisto- soma	Hookworm	Ascaris	Trichuris	Strongyloides
52.90***	−6.30	−3.91	−4.24	2.54	2.65
(3.45)	(5.72)	(3.83)	(3.83)	(4.02)	(9.20)

$R^2 = 0.022$; standard error $= 23.635$; $F_{7, 150} = 0.68$ (F $< 95\%$ level of significance).

Note: N = 158.
*** Significant at the .01 level (two-tailed test).

source of water for bathing, source of water for laundering, knowledge of germ theory, father's education, and father's occupation. This model can be expressed, therefore, in terms of the effects on pupils' achievement scores of region—including Castries and other urban areas—source of water for drinking, bathing, and laundering; knowledge of germ theory; parasite infection—including *Schistosoma,* hookworm, *Ascaris, Trichuris,* and *Strongyloides*—and parental socio-economic status, including father's education and occupation.

As shown in Table C.6, none of the parasitic infections are significant in explaining achievement scores. (The overall ability of this model to explain the variance in achievement, however, was much greater than the preceding model—the R^2 being 0.36 compared to 0.02.) A pupil's source of unsafe water for laundering had a negative association with test score, but unsafe water for bathing entered with a positive sign and was significant at the .05 level, indicating that pupils with more exposure to schistosomiasis via this activity actually achieved higher scores. This finding could be interpreted, perhaps, as indicating misspecification of our model; that is, the more "intelligent" pupils, perhaps being the more active and hence the more likely to use streams in bathing, may thereby

Table C.6. Additive Model Regression Coefficients (and Standard Errors), Reading Test Scores as Dependent Variable

			Source of water for			Knowledge of germ theory
Constant	Castries	Other urban	Drinking	Bathing	Launder-ing	
36.14**	28.71***	11.33**	−2.33	13.04**	−9.99*	−10.85***
(5.22)	(4.95)	(4.80)	(6.79)	(6.45)	(5.87)	(3.27)
		Parasite				
Schis-tosoma	Hook-worm	*Ascaris*	*Trich-uris*	*Strongy-loides*	Father's education	Father's occupation
−4.87	−0.81	0.79	2.31	6.38	5.06	11.64***
(4.91)	(3.81)	(3.37)	(3.40)	(7.75)	(3.40)	(4.47)

$R^2 = 0.364$; standard error $= 19.586$; $F_{13, 143} = 6.33$ (significance at 99% level requires $F > 2.15$).

Note: N = 158.
* Significant at the .10 level (two-tailed test).
** Significant at the .05 level (two-tailed test).
*** Significant at the .01 level (two-tailed test).

be more likely to contract schistosomiasis. The higher intelligence of these students might cancel out the effects of the disease so that infection is not shown to affect a pupil's performance.

Table C.7 tests whether the impact of parasitic infection varies with residence. The analysis includes three different formulations, with the top panel showing regression results for Castries schoolchildren, the middle panel showing the results for pupils in other urban areas, and the bottom panel showing the results for rural schoolchildren.

Our sample included few students who were infected with only one disease, and, in fact, included only two students with schistosomiasis alone. Therefore, we could not compare the effects of individual diseases with the effects of multiple diseases. However, using a somewhat different set of definitions for the disease variables, we can show that the effects of having more than one parasitic infection are less severe than the sum of the effects of the individual parasites. Table C.8 shows the results of linear regression (the order of variables in the equation corresponds to the order of t ratios, from highest to lowest) with the Nelson Reading Test score as the dependent variable and father's education, father's occupation, the combination of father's education and father's occupation, and all the parasites individually and in combination for which there were five or more observations, as the independent variables.

Table C.7. Additive Model Regression Coefficients (and Standard Errors), Showing Castries, Other Urban Areas, and Rural Schoolchildren, Reading Test Scores as Dependent Variable

| | Source of water for | | | Knowledge of germ theory | Parasite | | | | |
| | Drinking | Bathing | Laundering | | Schistosoma | Hookworm | Ascaris | Trichuris | Strongy-loides |
Constant									
Castries schoolchildren (N = 57)									
72.47***	-34.43	.00	8.21	-16.82***	-10.48	-3.43	-4.62	12.14*	-7.52
(7.24)	(27.93)	(19.41)	(21.70)	(5.93)	(8.46)	(6.55)	(6.12)	(6.41)	(12.00)

R² = 0.374; standard error = 19.198; $F_{11,45}$ = 2.74 (significance at 99% level requires F > 2.67).

| | Source of water for | | | Knowledge of germ theory | Parasite | | | | |
| | Drinking | Bathing | Laundering | | Schistosoma | Hookworm | Ascaris | Trichuris | Strongy-loides |
Constant									
Other urban schoolchildren (N = 58)									
45.91***	21.24	4.93	-18.94*	-3.91	-1.97	-1.09	-2.84	-3.39	26.40
(10.09)	(26.56)	(15.41)	(11.07)	(6.93)	(12.56)	(7.97)	(7.20)	(6.80)	(22.18)

R² = 0.252; standard error = 21.400; $F_{11,46}$ = 1.41 (F < 95% level of significance).

| | Source of water for | | | Knowledge of germ theory | Parasite | | | | |
| | Drinking | Bathing | Laundering | | Schistosoma | Hookworm | Ascaris | Trichuris | Strongy-loides |
Constant									
Rural schoolchildren (N = 43)									
28.31***	-5.13	8.72	1.15	-11.98**	-2.67	5.75	2.38	5.35	8.98
(6.28)	(6.47)	(7.05)	(7.66)	(5.25)	(7.64)	(6.45)	(5.20)	(5.57)	(10.68)

R² = 0.352; standard error = 15.997; $F_{11,31}$ = 1.53 (F < 95% level of significance).

 * Significant at the .10 level (two-tailed test).
 ** Significant at the .05 level (two-tailed test).
 *** Significant at the .01 level (two-tailed test).

Table C.8. Interaction Model Regression Coefficients (and Standard Errors), Aggregate Island-Wide Survey Data for Reading Test Scores as Dependent Variable

Independent variable*	Reading test scores
Constant	52.16***
	(5.31)
Father's education	11.91***
	(4.18)
Father's occupation	19.39*
	(11.11)
A, T	25.72***
	(9.18)
A	−18.52***
	(6.67)
T	−13.73**
	(6.62)
Father's education and	−15.08
father's occupation	(12.50)
H	−22.28**
	(10.35)
H, T	−21.89
	(13.56)
Sc	−24.16
	(23.21)
Sc, H	41.38
	(33.90)
H, A	33.14*
	(19.72)
H, A, T	−34.38
	(22.68)
Sc, H, T	−31.62
	(42.56)
Sc, T	20.45
	(25.40)
T, St	11.37
	(19.69)
St	−6.27
	(16.65)
Sc, A	14.88
	(26.97)
Sc, A, T	−11.60
	(31.37)
Sc, H, A, T	−10.52
	(31.33)
R^2	0.19
F ratio	1.69

Note: A = *Ascaris*, H = Hookworm, Sc = *Schistosoma*, St = *Strongyloides*, T = *Trichuris*.

  * Significant at the .10 level (two-tailed test).

  ** Significant at the .05 level (two-tailed test).

  *** Significant at the .01 level (two-tailed test).

The variables in this model differ from those in the other models in this volume that show interaction effects. To analyze the effect of a given combination-of-parasite variable in the present model, we must solve the regression equation not only for that variable but also for all elements of which it is composed. For example, taking only the one combination—*Ascaris* and *Trichuris*—that was significant at the .01 level (no other combination was significant at even the .05 level) we can predict a pupil's achievement, other things being equal, by summing the constant term, the coefficient for the interaction parasite variable—*Ascaris/Trichuris*—and the individual parasite variables—*Ascaris* and *Trichuris*. Hence, estimated achievement = 52.16 + 25.72 − 18.52 − 13.72 = 45.64. This sum is higher than the values predicted for the simple additive effects of *Ascaris* and *Trichuris* (achievement = 52.16 − 18.52 − 13.72 = 19.92) and even for each of the individual parasites alone (for *Ascaris*, achievement = 52.16 − 18.52 = 33.64, and for *Trichuris*, achievement = 52.16 − 13.72 = 38.44).

This shows that having two parasites is associated with having a higher achievement score than having only one parasite. This finding may seem implausible, in that it may be interpreted as stating that contracting a second parasitic infection actually *raises* the level of achievement. This could occur, however, if the multiple parasites interacted in such a way as to diminish the vitality of the parasites individually. In addition, of course, our findings may simply reflect an inability to control for all relevant variables—biological and other.

Table C.9 shows, for the Babonneau school study—in an area of high prevalence of schistosomiasis—the mean and standard deviation for each variable and for several combinations-of-parasite variables. The latter are included so as to determine whether effects of diseases interact and, hence, if the effects of having more than one parasitic infection are not simply additive. In this analysis we concentrated attention on *Schistosoma* and the possible effects of other parasites in combination with *Schistosoma*, without distinguishing among the other parasites. Thus, we included (dummy) variables for *Schistosoma*-plus-one-other parasite, *Schistosoma*-plus-two-other parasites, and *Schistosoma*-plus-three-other parasites.

It is noteworthy that although more than half of the 267 children sampled were free of schistosomiasis, no youngster in the sample was free of all four parasitic infections. As a result, the data preclude comparison of infected children with children whose level of health was excellent, in the sense of their being uninfected with any parasite.

Our hypothesis once again is that schistosomiasis, alone or in combination with other parasitic diseases, exerts a *negative* effect on the child's

Table C.9. Means and Standard Deviations of Variables Used in the Babonneau School Survey

Variable	Mean	Standard deviation
Weight (pounds)	73.022	15.740
Height (inches)	54.551	3.879
Class rank (100 minus actual rank)[a]	83.730	10.115
Number of days absent during year	23.809	20.028
Schistosoma (1 if present, 0 if not)	0.401	0.491
Hookworm (1 if present, 0 if not)	0.581	0.494
Ascaris (1 if present, 0 if not)	0.543	0.499
Trichuris (1 if present, 0 if not)	0.700	0.461
Egg count (Schistosome eggs/gram)	24.816	73.694
Age (years)	11.963	1.620
Sex (1 if male, 0 if female)	0.491	0.501
Schistosoma & one other parasite (1 if *Schistosoma* and only one other parasite present, 0 otherwise)	0.150	0.358
Schistosoma & two other parasites (1 if *Schistosoma* and only two other parasites present, 0 otherwise)	0.135	0.342
Schistosoma & three other parasites (1 if all four parasites present, 0 otherwise)	0.060	0.238

Note: N = 267.

[a] Actual rank was subtracted from a constant—arbitrarily 100—in order that a student who was near the top of the class would have a high class rank.

vitality (as measured by absenteeism), physical condition (as measured by height and weight), and, eventually, academic achievement (as measured by class rank). We recognize, though, that causation may actually be in both directions; not only may disease affect performance and physical condition, but the likelihood that a child is infected by parasites may depend on how active he is physically—how often he is out playing in schistosomiasis-infested streams or running around barefoot on hookworm-infested ground—and how much he has learned about means of avoiding disease. Thus, we do not rule out the possibility of observing significant *positive* relationships between our dependent variables and the "independent," disease variables.[3] Such findings, while inconsistent with the hypothesis that schistosomiasis and the other parasitic diseases exert a *strong* negative effect, would not preclude existence of a relatively *weak* negative effect. Such a weak effect could be swamped by the offsetting effect of variation among children in their "natural" levels of motivation to learn in school, to play in streams and so forth—variation for which it was not possible to control explicitly.

Table C.10. Additive and Interaction Models Regression Coefficients (and Standard Errors), Babonneau School Survey, Weight as Dependent Variable

Constant	Age	Sex	*Schistosoma*	Schistosome egg count	Hookworm	*Ascaris*	*Trichuris*
−4.64	6.59***	−5.30***	−.71	0.01	0.61	−1.53	2.70*
(5.50)	(0.42)	(1.37)	(1.51)	(0.01)	(1.43)	(1.40)	(1.52)

$R^2 = 0.512$; standard error = 11.145 pounds; $F_{7,\,259} = 38.80$ (significance at 99% level requires $F > 2.70$).

Constant	Age	Sex	*Schistosoma*	Schistosome egg count	*Schistosoma* & one other parasite	*Schistosoma* & two other parasites	*Schistosoma* & three other parasites
−4.13	6.67***	−5.33***	−3.36	0.01	2.30	4.08	1.36
(5.28)	(0.43)	(1.39)	(3.05)	(0.01)	(3.40)	(3.45)	(4.06)

$R^2 = 0.506$; standard error = 11.214 pounds; $F_{7,\,259} = 37.86$ (significance at 99% level requires $F > 2.70$).

Note: N = 267.
    * Indicates significance at the .10 level (two-tailed test).
    *** Indicates significance at the .01 level (two-tailed test).

Tables C.10–C.13 show the results of ordinary least-squares linear regressions in which the dependent variables are, in turn, the student's weight (Table C.10), the student's height (Table C.11), the number of days absent from school (Table C.12), and the student's class rank (Table C.13). The analysis employs two alternative formulations: in the top panel of each table the parasite variables were entered separately; in the bottom panel the possibility of interaction effects among parasites was

3. We recall that in our island-wide survey, pupils who used streams or irrigation canals in which to bathe actually performed better on tests than users of safe water. Yet we found no significant relationship between use of hazardous sources of water for bathing and schistosomiasis infection.

Table C.11. Additive and Interaction Models Regression Coefficients (and Standard Errors), Babonneau School Survey, Height as Dependent Variable

Constant	Age	Sex	Schis- tosoma	Schis- tosome egg count	Hook- worm	Ascaris	Trichuris
35.86***	1.55***	−0.51	−0.35	−0.001	0.28	−0.19	0.72*
(1.45)	(0.11)	(0.36)	(0.40)	(0.003)	(0.38)	(0.37)	(0.40)

$R^2 = 0.442$; standard error = 2.938 inches; $F_{7, 259} = 29.26$ (significance at 99% level requires $F > 2.70$).

Constant	Age	Sex	Schis- tosoma	Schis- tosome egg count	Schis- tosoma & one other parasite	Schis- tosoma & two other parasites	Schis- tosoma & three other parasites
36.59***	1.54***	−0.47	−1.43*	−0.002	1.03	0.88	1.87*
(1.39)	(0.11)	(0.36)	(0.80)	(0.003)	(0.89)	(0.91)	(1.07)

$R^2 = 0.439$; standard error = 2.945 inches; $F_{7, 259} = 28.92$ (significance at 99% level requires $F > 2.70$).

Note: N = 267.
  * Indicates significance at the .10 level (two-tailed test).
  *** Indicates significance at the .01 level (two-tailed test).

Table C.12. Additive and Interaction Models Regression Coefficients (and Standard Errors), Babonneau School Survey, Days Absent as Dependent Variable

Con- stant	Age	Sex	Schistosoma	Schis- tosome egg count	Hook- worm	Ascaris	Trichuris
6.53	1.09	6.24***	−3.37	0.001	3.12	2.60	−0.83
(9.72)	(0.75)	(2.43)	(2.68)	(0.017)	(2.54)	(2.48)	(2.70)

$R^2 = 0.057$; standard error = 19.714 days; $F_{7, 259} = 2.22$ (significance at 95% level requires $F > 2.05$).

Con- stant	Age	Sex	Schistosoma	Schis- tosome egg count	Schis- tosoma & one other parasite	Schis- tosoma & two other parasites	Schis- tosoma & three other parasites
9.00	1.13	6.16***	−11.81**	0.002	7.40	11.47*	5.07
(9.26)	(0.76)	(2.43)	(5.35)	(0.017)	(5.97)	(6.04)	(7.12)

$R^2 = 0.062$; standard error = 19.661 days; $F_{7, 259} = 2.43$ (significance at 95% level requires $F > 2.05$).

Note: N = 267.
  * Indicates significance at the .10 level (two-tailed test).
  ** Indicates significance at the .05 level (two-tailed test).
  *** Indicates significance at the .01 level (two-tailed test).

Table C.13. Additive and Interaction Models Regression Coefficients (and Standard Errors), Babonneau School Survey, Class Rank as Dependent Variable

Constant	Sex	*Schistosoma*	Schistosome egg count	Hookworm	*Ascaris*	*Trichuris*
84.09***	−3.04***	1.16	−0.01	1.32	0.70	−0.27
(1.86)	(1.24)	(1.36)	(0.01)	(1.29)	(1.26)	(1.37)

$R^2 = 0.034$; standard error $= 10.054$; $F_{6,\ 260} = 1.54$ (significance at 90% level requires $F > 1.75$).

Constant	Sex	*Schistosoma*	Schistosome egg count	*Schistosoma* & one other parasite	*Schistosoma* & two other parasites	*Schistosoma* & three other parasites
85.14***	−2.95***	−1.54	−0.01	2.39	2.63	3.60
(1.04)	(1.24)	(2.73)	(0.01)	(3.05)	(3.09)	(3.62)

$R^2 = 0.034$; standard error $= 10.058$; $F_{6,\ 260} = 1.51$ (significance at 90% level requires $F > 1.75$).

Note: $N = 267$. A positive association between an independent variable and class rank indicates that an increase in the value of the variable is associated with an improvement in class rank.

*** Indicates significance at the .01 level (two-tailed test).

explored by entering as separate variables combinations of other parasites with *Schistosoma*. The latter formulation as with all of our other interaction models, was included to explore the possibility that a person who has, say, schistosomiasis and hookworm will be more (or perhaps less) sick than he would be if he had each of the two parasitic infections "separately." Thus, this model can be thought of as testing for the presence of increasing or decreasing "returns"—impacts—to the number of diseases. Table C.14 is the zero order correlation matrix for these Babonneau school studies.

As a further test for interaction effects among parasites, linear regressions were estimated for a model including all but one of the fifteen possible combinations of the four parasites for which data were available, in addition to age and sex. Since no student in the sample was free of all four parasites it was necessary to exclude one parasite variable. It was decided to exclude *Ascaris* (alone), since a priori indications were that it had the smallest effects.

Our interest in the effects of parasitic infection on *achievement* in school led us to focus on absences and class rank as key dependent variables. The results (shown in Table C.15) disclosed that none of the fourteen parasite

Table C.14. Matrix of Correlation Coefficients, Babonneau School Survey

	Hookworm	Ascaris	Trichuris	Egg count	Age	Sex	Weight	Height	Class rank	Days absent	Schistosoma & one other parasite	Schistosoma & two other parasites	Schistosoma & three other parasites
Schistosoma	-.23	-.17	-.16	.26	-.02	-.10	-.01	-.02	.03	-.12	.51	.48	.31
Hookworm		-.05	.13	-.02	.03	.08	.04	.07	.01	.10	-.28	.02	.22
Ascaris			.02	-.09	-.06	-.02	-.09	-.05	.03	.07	-.20	-.01	.23
Trichuris				-.16	.02	-.00	.08	.11	.00	.01	-.22	.14	.17
Egg count					.08	.00	.10	.00	-.07	.02	.25	.06	.00
Age						.00	.67	.65	-.08	.07	.00	-.09	.11
Sex							-.16	-.06	-.15	.17	-.08	.01	-.09
Weight								.85	-.09	.02	.01	-.03	.07
Height									-.06	.10	-.02	-.10	.12
Class rank										-.10	.01	.02	.06
Days absent											-.06	.02	-.07
Schistosoma & one other parasite												-.17	-.11
Schistosoma & two other parasites													-.10

Table C.15. Interaction Model Regression Coefficients (and Standard Errors), Babonneau School Survey, Absences and Class Rank as Dependent Variables

Independent variable	Dependent variable	
	Days absent	Class rank
Constant	8.7	84.2***
	(10.6)	(2.6)
Age	1.05	—
	(0.76)	
Sex	5.39**	−2.40*
(0 if female; 1 if male)	(2.46)	(1.24)
T	−4.64	1.37
	(7.16)	(3.62)
A, T	1.98	3.53
	(6.52)	(3.28)
H	9.31	1.84
	(7.45)	(3.76)
H, T	−3.51	−2.11
	(6.09)	(3.07)
H, A	10.20	−3.87
	(7.82)	(3.94)
H, A, T	3.54	1.37
	(5.80)	(2.92)
Sc	−10.18	−1.40
	(7.17)	(3.61)
Sc, T	−1.04	−3.19
	(6.86)	(3.46)
Sc, A	−8.57	2.93
	(7.64)	(3.84)
Sc, A, T	3.08	−3.50
	(7.32)	(3.68)
Sc, H	1.07	5.25
	(8.01)	(4.04)
Sc, H, T	0.87	5.44
	(6.96)	(3.51)
Sc, H, A	−2.28	0.71
	(10.14)	(5.11)
Sc, H, A, T	−5.18	2.50
	(7.07)	(3.56)
R^2	0.10	0.10
F ratio	1.71	1.78

Note: A = *Ascaris*, H = Hookworm, Sc = *Schistosoma*, T = *Trichuris*.
  * Significant at the .10 level (two-tailed test).
  ** Significant at the .05 level (two-tailed test).
  *** Significant at the .01 level (two-tailed test).

variables, singly or in combination, had an effect on either dependent variable that was significantly different from zero at anywhere near even the .10 level. Again it might be noted that no data were available on the *intensity* of any parasite except *Schistosoma*, and even for that infection, the egg-count—the reliability of which is subject to debate in medical circles—was available for only a relatively small number of pupils.

Appendix D

TECHNICAL DISCUSSION OF THE LABOR PRODUCTIVITY ANALYSIS

As described in chapter 5, we tested four hypotheses relating the presence of parasitic infection to labor productivity. In addition to the main hypothesis (1) that infection leads to reduced earnings, we also tested three others that underlie it: infected workers, as gauged by the presence of parasites in their bodies, work at jobs that are physically less demanding (hypothesis 2); they are less productive per day worked on any given type of work (hypothesis 3); and they work fewer days per week—that is, are absent more from the job (hypothesis 4).[1]

Figure D.1 illustrates these possibilities by comparing hypothetical supply and demand functions for a typical "sick" and a typical "healthy" worker who are identical in all other relevant respects—the amount and quality of capital and land with which each works, their education levels, age, etc.—except for disease. Since it is expected that healthy workers will supply more labor at any given wage rate, the supply curve of the healthy worker, S_H, is drawn to the right of the supply curve of the sick worker. Thus, at the wage rate OC, for example, the sick worker supplies only CE

---

1. We noted in chapter 5 that days per week—rather than days per month or per year—were selected as the dependent variable in testing the relationship between illnesses and labor supply because medical examinations and interviews suggested that most of any effects of disease on the labor supply would manifest themselves in this variable. Factors difficult to quantify are likely to be significant in accounting for differences in weeks worked per month or year.

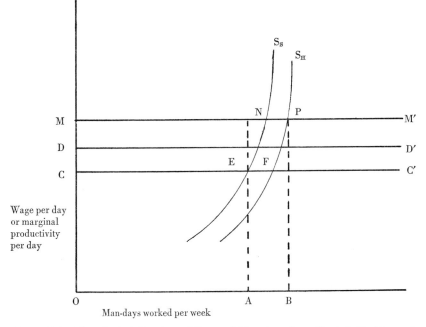

Figure D.1. Hypothetical Supply and Demand Functions for a Typical Healthy and a Typical Sick Worker

days of work per week whereas the healthy worker supplies CF days per week on this job. The greater productivity of healthy workers compared with sick workers on the same job is indicated by drawing the marginal productivity curve for the healthy worker, DD', above that of the sick worker, CC'.[2] MM' is the healthy worker's marginal productivity on another, higher productivity job.

The demand (marginal productivity) and supply curves are drawn as if the four hypotheses specified above hold. (1) The typical healthy person's total earnings—represented by the area OMPB—are greater than

2. The horizontal shape of the marginal productivity curves reflects the assumptions that increasing the number of days worked per week for an individual (or even for a relatively small group) has a negligible effect in reducing the capital/labor and land/labor ratios and that each laborer works equally hard each day regardless of the number of days per week he spends on the job. The greater marginal productivity of healthy workers may be due not only to their ability to work harder on any given job but also their ability to undertake more physically demanding and productive jobs, for example, "task" work versus "day" work. The line MM' indicates the marginal productivity level of a healthy worker on a more productive job than represented by DD' or CC'.

those of a sick person's—shown by the area OCEA; (2) the job depicted by the marginal productivity curve CC' for the sick worker, and DD' for the healthy worker is physically less demanding than the job represented by MM'; (3) the marginal productivity per day of a sick person on this less-demanding job OC, which is less than that of a healthy person on the same job, is assumed to be OD; and (4) average sick employees work fewer days per week than average healthy employees, that is, OA is less than OB. CC' is, in effect, the demand for sick workers, while MM' is the demand for healthy workers.

The methodology employed below is to compare (a) the labor supply, and (b) the productivity of workers who are similar in all important respects except that they vary in conditions of health. Specifically, hypothesis 1—disease reduces weekly earnings—will be tested by regressing *earnings per week* on a number of disease and other personal characteristic variables. Hypothesis 2—disease causes workers to shift to physically less-demanding jobs—will be tested by regressing the ratio of days worked at *task* jobs to *total* days worked (over an eighteen-month period) on the same independent variables used in testing hypothesis 1. This ratio reflects the judgment that task work—including such work as digging drainage canals and carrying bananas from the field—is more difficult than day work (per dollar earned) ; hence, we expect that ill workers will do relatively less task work. Hypothesis 3—disease reduces productivity per day—will be tested by regressing earnings per day from all types of work, on the independent variables, as well as by regressing earnings and output per day for each of four different task jobs on these same independent variables. Finally, hypothesis 4—disease reduces the amount of labor supplied per week—will be tested by regressing days worked per week on the independent variables.

Our expectations are that statistically significant negative coefficients for the disease variables will be found for all four hypotheses. We recognize, however, that, with respect to hypothesis 4, a positive income effect may attenuate or even reverse the negative effect of poor health.

There is another reason for possibly finding a positive relationship, rather than the expected negative relationship, between disease and days worked per week (hypothesis 4), as well as between disease and earnings per day (hypothesis 3) and between disease and the percentage of days worked at task jobs. People who work more or harder and who work around infested water or infested soil are more likely to contract parasitic diseases. Once again we see that identification of "independent" and "dependent" variables is not simple, since causation may run in two directions—in this case, from labor effort to disease prevalence, as well as in the opposite direction. It is quite possible that, even though a disease reduces the daily productivity (earnings) of the more energetic workers and also the average number of days they work per week, average weekly earnings of these workers may still be higher than for the rest of the labor force. Because it has not been possible to account completely for differences in physical ability, motivation, and work-preference patterns among workers, the cross-sectional analysis utilized here might not in this case show the detrimental effect of sickness on either actual or potential productivity. Thus, although in any of the regressions testing hypotheses 1, 2, 3, or 4 we will regard negative coefficients as being consistent with the specific hypotheses, we must be cautious before rejecting the hypotheses on the basis of positive coefficients, for we are unable to specify and estimate the model of productivity determination in a fully satisfactory way.

The results from testing the model just outlined must be used very carefully when estimating the output effects of improving health conditions for *all* workers in St. Lucia. The reason is that any significant change in the number of man-days of labor supplied—such as may result from a substantial improvement in health[3]—would mean, at least in the short run, a decrease in the capital/labor and land/labor ratios and, therefore, a decline in the productivity of (healthy) labor. It is possible, therefore, as was pointed out in chapter 1, that the marginal productivity and earnings per day of labor, and even the average level of weekly earnings, as well as aggregate labor earnings, could decline as a result of the improvement in health conditions. Workers could be worse off financially.

But the extreme result of an actual reduction in total labor income resulting from an improvement in health which increases the supply of labor is that the marginal-revenue-product-of-labor function for the economy has an elasticity of between 0 and -1, in the relevant range. In such a case, improved health would raise *total* output (the area under the marginal-product-of-labor curve) but would actually reduce the absolute size of *labor's share*. This outcome appears to be unlikely in St. Lucia, however. Based on our knowledge of the production function for bananas and the foreign demand for St. Lucian bananas, our impression is that the marginal-revenue-product function for labor is quite elastic. Total wage income is not likely to decline as a result of an improvement in health conditions.

One possibly important limitation of our data should be noted. Because

3. As noted, it is possible that better health causes an individual to reduce, rather than increase, his labor supply because of a strong income effect associated with the increase in his earnings per day. However, an offset to this possible negative supply effect in the economy is the probable entrance into the labor force of workers who previously were too sick to work. This assumes that the parasitic infections are severe enough, at least in some meaningful number of cases, to keep workers out of the labor force.

the data apply to workers who were actually employed, persons who were severely disabled by disease would not have been observed; they would either be too weak to offer their labor or would be insufficiently productive or dependable to be retained by an employer. As a result there is a priori reason to believe that our findings as to the overall labor supply and productivity effects of disease are biased; the true effects over the entire range of disease severity may well be greater than those observed among *employed* workers. This bias is analogous to a possible bias in the scholastic-performance study, where it was pointed out that if there were any seriously debilitated youngsters they would also be missing from the sample, either because they were too ill to attend school at all or because they died during the period. (Appendix F is devoted to the question of the representativeness of our data samples.) The omission of extreme severe cases, though, is unlikely to affect the algebraic sign or statistical significance of the relationships we estimate between parasitic infection and our various behavior measures. A person with even a severe schistosomiasis infection is not likely *suddenly* to become so incapacitated that he cannot work (or attend school). Rather, the expectation is that he *gradually* becomes weaker until finally, in the most extreme cases, he may be unable to work. Thus, we would expect to find that workers who are infected with parasites but are still able to work to some extent would be less vigorous and less productive than healthier workers.

Hypothesis 1: Earnings Per Week

Little is known about the manner in which the disease variables influence labor effort. Therefore, in order to permit a maximum degree of flexibility we included a (dummy) variable for each of the five parasites singly and also in combination with each other, in order to permit interdependencies to show up if they were present. The various personal characteristics of the workers that were described in the last section are also included in the model for the purpose of isolating the disease effects. Equation (1) summarizes this broad model of the determinants of the average earnings per week for various groups of Geest workers.

(1) $W = a_0 + (a_1, a_2, \ldots, a_{31}) [D] + a_{32}LS + a_{33}M + a_{34}P + a_{35}Y + a_{36}Y^2 + a_{37}E + a_{38}NGW + a_{39}GB + a_{40}GH,$

where W = mean earnings per week;

$[D]$ = a row vector (1×31) of dummy variables of the thirty-one possible combinations of the five parasitic infections;[4]

4. Tests of significance for the differences between the means of the different variables for the entire sample and for the various subsamples indicate that the subsamples are representative of the entire sample.

LS and M = dummy variables indicating whether the individual
does, 1, or does not, 0, have an enlarged liver or
spleen (LS) or a low hemoglobin count (M); all
of these are symptoms of severe schistosomiasis infection, but also are symptoms of other diseases;

P = number of pregnancies during lifetime (used only
in analyzing the female group);

Y and Y^2 = years of age and age squared;

E = years of schooling; and

NGW, GB, and GH = dummy variables reflecting whether the individual
does, 1, or does not, 0, work for any employer in addition to Geest (that is, whether he does any non-
Geest work—NGW); does or does not grow bananas
himself (GB); and does or does not live in Geest-
owned (somewhat higher quality) housing (GH).

Negative coefficients were expected for the *disease variables* and for
their symptoms, liver and spleen enlargement and low hemoglobin count,
although, as pointed out above, positive coefficients are not absolutely inconsistent with the occurrence of debilitating effects of disease. *Number
of pregnancies* was used as a proxy measure for the number of a woman's
dependents, and, hence, was expected to have a negative coefficient. *Age*
was expected to exert a positive effect on earnings up to some age beyond
which a negative effect was anticipated; the inclusion of variables for
both age and age squared permitted testing for such an age effect, as had
been found in the demographic work above. *Amount of education,* E, was
included primarily to reflect skill and motivation; a positive sign was
hypothesized. *Working for an employer in addition to Geest,* NGW, and
growing one's own bananas, GB, were both intended to reflect work effort
devoted to other activities, and so negative signs were expected. The
variable reflecting whether a worker lived in *Geest housing,* GH, was included to control for the possible effects of this somewhat better than
average quality housing, and also for its relative proximity to the place
of work, both of which might be expected to be associated with greater
number of days worked—that is, with positive coefficients. The values of
the means and standard deviations for a selection of these variables from
some of the regression models are given in Table D.1.

As a practical matter equation (1) could not be estimated because the
sample data included no observations for many of the thirty-one combinations of parasitic infections, and only a few observations for others. Therefore, we actually estimated equation (1) as modified to include only the
combination of disease variables for which there were at least five ob-

Table D.1. Means and Standard Deviations of Selected Variables Used in the Geest Agricultural-Worker Studies

Variable	Table number[a]	Mean		Standard deviation	
		Male	Female	Male	Female
Age	D.2	41.61	36.40	12.28	14.29
Education (years)	D.2	1.73	1.60	2.95	3.04
Non-Geest work, proportion doing	D.2	.73	.43	.45	.50
Pregnancies during lifetime	D.2	—	4.45	—	2.64
Geest housing, proportion having	D.2	.22	.32	.42	.47
Grow own bananas, proportion	D.2	.16	.17	.37	.38
Sc, H, A, proportion having	D.2	.24	.10	.43	.30
Sc, H, A, T, proportion having	D.2	.22	.33	.42	.48
Sc, proportion having	D.3 (Qual. model)	.82	.67	.39	.48
H, proportion having	D.3	.94	.92	.24	.28
A, proportion having	D.3	.64	.72	.48	.45
T, proportion having	D.3	.40	.58	.49	.50
St, proportion having	D.3	.27	.13	.45	.34

Note: A = *Ascaris*, H = Hookworm, Sc = *Schistosoma*, St = *Strongyloides*, T = *Trichuris*. Means and standard deviations for variables in other tables are available from the authors.

[a] The table number reference identifies the particular regression model for which the means and standard deviations presented here were calculated.

servations—an arbitrary number that had previously been set so as to achieve "reasonable" sample size. The results, in Table D.2, show that not one of the combinations of parasitic infections—six for men and four for women—was statistically significant in explaining variations in workers' earnings per week.[5]

Another useful way of analyzing the effects of the disease variables is to assume that there is a simple additive relationship between each parasitic infection and the dependent variable. This implies estimating the equation:

(2) $W = a_0 + a_1Sc + a_2H + a_3A + a_4T + a_5St +$ all other nondisease variables included in (1).

5. The effect of omitting several of the disease combinations is to include these combinations in the constant term. Thus the disease combinations explicitly included are to be interpreted relative to the average effect of those diseases on the constant term.

Table D.2. Interaction Model Regression Coefficients (and Standard Errors), Geest Worker Earnings Per Week as Dependent Variable

Independent variable	Coefficients (and standard errors)	
	Males (N = 50) (1)	Females (N = 60) (2)
Constant	−339 (587)	141 (256)
Age	50 (30)	17 (12)
Age squared	−.59 (.36)	−0.20 (0.14)
Education (years)	−28 (21)	6 (12)
Non-Geest work	−52 (154)	54 (68)
Pregnancies, number of	—	19 (16)
Geest housing	175 (161)	11 (77)
Grow own bananas	−140 (175)	9 (15)
H	—	−68 (119)
Sc, H	189 (242)	—
Sc, H, A	26 (223)	−20 (125)
Sc, H, A, T	−113 (230)	−57 (83)
H, A	116 (268)	—
H, A, T	—	−97 (118)
Sc, H, T	8 (265)	—
Sc, H, T, St	−0.3 (245)	—
R^2	.25	.13
F ratio	1.10	.63

Note: A = *Ascaris*, H = Hookworm, Sc = *Schistosoma*, St = *Strongyloides*, T = *Trichuris*. Dashes indicate insufficient observations. None of the coefficients in the table are significant at the .10 level (two-tailed test).

In this formulation, a person who has, say, schistosomiasis and hook-worm, would be included both among persons having Sc and also among persons having H, whereas in equation (1) a person indicated as having Sc had that and only that disease.

Table D.3. Additive Models Regression Coefficients (and Standard Errors), Geest Worker Earnings Per Week as Dependent Variable

| | Coefficients (and standard errors) | | | |
| Independent variable | Qualitative model | | Quantitative model | |
	Males (N = 66) (1)	Females (N = 59) (2)	Males (N = 45) (3)	Females (N = 23) (4)
Constant	286 (554)	29 (284)	206 (518)	3 (318)
Schistosoma	−105 (146)	2 (80)		
Few eggs			−144 (143)	24 (118)
Many eggs			20 (141)	−54 (99)
Hookworm	−41 (205)	40 (119)	−86 (120)	—
Ascaris	−125 (105)	−42 (85)	−87 (117)	−163 (108)
Trichuris	−69 (103)	−18 (73)	58 (113)	26 (118)
Strongyloides	−2 (127)	148 (102)	—	−305*** (101)
Age	20 (24)	19 (12)	28 (25)	44*** (16)
Age squared	−0.2 (0.3)	−0.24 (0.14)	−.37 (.30)	−0.50*** (0.19)
Education (years)	−24 (17)	8 (11)	−14 (20)	−9 (12)
Non-Geest work	70 (125)	60 (69)	25 (137)	20 (113)
Geest housing	108 (133)	46 (79)	133 (145)	−45 (104)
Grow own bananas	−112 (135)	14 (15)	−164 (149)	−0.1 (195)
Pregnancies		22 (16)		0.2 (1.5)
R²	0.16	0.16	0.19	0.67
F ratio	0.94	0.74	0.72	1.89

Note: Dashes indicate insufficient observations.

  *** Significant at the .01 level (two-tailed test).

Table D.3 contains the estimates of equation (2) for males and for females. The variables indicating liver or spleen enlargement and low hemoglobin count have been dropped, because in addition to having been found in test regressions to be insignificant, the information about them is not available for a sizable number of workers; as a result their inclusion would have further reduced what was already a modest sample size.

The absence of statistical significance in equation (1) of the disease variables has another implication. Pairwise, comparison of parasite combinations that differ by only one parasite—for example, Sc, H and Sc, H, A for males in column 1, Table D.2—discloses that the coefficients are not significantly different from each other; thus, for example, the addition of *Ascaris*, A, to the combination of *Schistosoma* and hookworm, Sc, H, is not associated with a significant change in the coefficient. The difference between 189 (the coefficient of Sc, H) and 26 (the coefficient of Sc, H, A) is indeed less than the standard error of either of the two regression coefficients.

The four additive regressions in Table D.3 also fail to disclose any significant association of individual parasitic infection with weekly earnings, except that the quantitative model, in which the intensity of schistosomiasis is indicated by whether the person examined had "few" eggs (up to nineteen per gram) or "many," showed that one parasite, *Strongyloides*, appeared to exert a highly significant negative effect on the earnings of women (column 4). The difference between the "quantitative" regressions, columns 3 and 4, and the "qualitative" regressions, columns 1 and 2, is that the latter simply contain information on the presence or absence of schistosomal infection while the former contain a count of the number of schistosome eggs, as explained above.

An interesting question is whether the various parasites *as a group* have a significant depressing effect on earnings, under the assumption that their individually insignificant effects are additive. One test for this would be to perform an F-test for all the disease variables in those regressions in which each of the parasite-infection coefficients was negative, even though insignificant. Interpretation of the F-test for all diseases would be confusing when some of the disease coefficients were positive and others negative. In Table D.3, column 1, the necessary condition was met; analysis of the sample of sixty-six male agricultural workers disclosed that each of the five parasites exerted a negative effect on weekly earnings. Hence, we determined the F ratio for this study. Our finding was a ratio of 2.57, a value that is statistically significant at the .05 level. The total effect on weekly earnings of the entire group of parasitic infections is significantly negative, even though no individual disease has a significant negative effect.

Hypothesis 2: Task versus Day Work

To test our hypothesis that infected workers adjust to debility by choosing to do less task work than do uninfected workers,[6] the dependent variable

Table D.4. Additive Model Regression Coefficients (and Standard Errors), Geest Workers, Task-Days Worked as Percentage of Total Days Worked as Dependent Variable[a]

Independent variable	Coefficients (and standard errors)	
	Males (N = 35) (1)	Females (N = 23) (2)
Constant	0.17	.43
	(.21)	(0.29)
Schistosoma		
Few eggs	−0.003	−0.05
	(0.058)	(0.11)
Many eggs	−0.04	0.008
	(0.06)	(0.090)
Ascaris	−0.04	0.06
	(0.05)	(0.10)
Trichuris	0.006	−0.07
	(0.046)	(0.11)
Hookworm	−0.009	—
	(0.049)	
Strongyloides	—	−0.06
		(0.09)
Age	−0.003	−0.004
	(0.010)	(0.014)
Age squared	0.000	−0.000
	(.000)	(0.000)
Education	−0.009	0.01
	(0.008)	(0.01)
Non-Geest work	−0.04	−0.03
	(0.05)	(0.10)
Pregnancies		0.001
		(0.001)
Geest housing	−0.03	0.02
	(0.05)	(0.09)
Grow own bananas	0.05	−.11
	(0.06)	(.18)
R^2	.15	.44
F ratio	.54	.71

Note: Dashes indicate insufficient observations. None of the coefficients in the table are significant at the .10 level (two-tailed test).

[a] For persons performing task jobs on at least 10 percent of the days worked.

6. To take account of the possibility that occasionally a worker may be pressed into task work at peak work periods and also the possibility that the effect of

used was the proportion of days of task work to total days worked for each individual, while the independent variables were the same as those used in testing hypothesis 1. Estimates are in Table D.4 separately for males and females.[7]

Hypothesis 3: Productivity Per Day

If schistosomiasis and the other parasitic diseases cause debility among workers, another manner in which this might manifest itself is through effects on the workers' marginal productivity per day. A number of dependent variables were used to test for this relationship: earnings per day for all types of day and task work, taken as a whole, and earnings per day for four selected specific task jobs. The independent variables were the same as those employed in testing the other hypotheses.

Table D.5 indicates that schistosomiasis was associated with lower daily earnings for males, whereas *Strongyloides* was significantly related to lower earnings for females. As we pointed out in chapter 5, the indicated effect of schistosomiasis infection is a reduction of about 80 cents of earnings per day.

Table D.6 reveals, as noted in chapter 5, that among males performing tasks 1 and 3, those men who also grew their own bananas earned significantly more per day worked for Geest. In the discussion following equation (1), above, it was predicted that Geest workers who also grew their own bananas would have *lower* earnings per *week*. This is, of course, perfectly consistent with the point being made here, that such workers are expected to have *higher* earnings per *day worked* for Geest. The fact that they grow their own bananas means that they work for Geest fewer days per week, on an average.

Hypothesis 4: Days Worked

Hypothesis 4—that the number of days worked would be reduced by the effects of disease—was investigated by regressing the average number of days worked per week (during the eighteen-month period) on the diseases and other independent variables. The results are shown in Table D.7.

---

disease on workers' stamina is negligible over very low ranges of task work, the sample is restricted to those who have performed task work on at least 10 percent of the days they have worked.

7. In reporting the results of this (and subsequent hypotheses), only the results of the additive regression model are presented; the interaction model, while having considerable appeal a priori, did not prove to be of great value, partly because the limited sample size produced a sizable number of combinations of diseases for which there were few if any observations.

Table D.5. Additive Model Regression Coefficients (and Standard Errors), Geest Workers, Earnings Per Day Worked as Dependent Variable

Independent variable	Coefficients (and standard errors)	
	Males (N = 45) (1)	Females (N = 23) (2)
Constant	522***	101*
	(151)	(51)
Schistosoma		
Few eggs	−86**	13
	(42)	(19)
Many eggs	−80*	−4
	(41)	(16)
Ascaris	10	−8
	(34)	(17)
Trichuris	−10	8
	(33)	(19)
Hookworm	−8	—
	(35)	
Strongyloides	—	−31*
		(16)
Age	−8	6.4***
	(7)	(2.5)
Age squared	0.07	−0.08**
	(0.09)	(0.03)
Education	−1	−2
	(6)	(2)
Non-Geest work	−63*	8
	(40)	(18)
Pregnancies		0.03
		(0.24)
Geest housing	−35	−3
	(42)	(17)
Grow own bananas	50	−11
	(44)	(31)
R^2	0.30	0.51
F ratio	1.34	0.95

Note: Dashes indicate insufficient observations.
 * Significant at the .10 level (two-tailed test).
 ** Significant at the .05 level (two-tailed test).
 *** Significant at the .01 level (two-tailed test).

le D.6. Additive Model Regression Coefficients (and Standard Errors), Geest Workers, nings Per Day on Specific Task Jobs as Dependent Variable

	Coefficients (and standard errors)					
	Task 1[a]		Task 2[b]	Task 3[c]		Task 4[d]
Independent variable	Females (N = 35) (1)	Males (N = 34) (2)	Females (N = 23) (3)	Males (N = 47) (4)	Females (N = 41) (5)	Males (N = 29) (6)
stant	435***	873	348	653	316***	776
	(115)	(563)	(233)	(1297)	(59)	(542)
stosoma	−43	64	34	−71	32.1*	−69
	(35)	(275)	(72)	(228)	(16.5)	(106)
aris	−68*	−517*	33	−353*	−10	−145
	(37)	(274)	(66)	(197)	(17)	(145)
huris	67**	−55	−33	103	−6	119
	(33)	(332)	(48)	(213)	(15)	(102)
kworm	−83	370	−22	160	39	−185
	(93)	(427)	(61)	(249)	(25)	(149)
ngyloides	−30	341	−75	134	−30	−56
	(51)	(420)	(59)	(255)	(22)	(139)
e	3	−21	−2	−3	0.1	9
	(6)	(32)	(13)	(69)	(3.0)	(32)
squared	−0.05	−0.4	0.05	−0.06	0.01	−0.08
	(0.07)	(0.6)	(0.20)	(0.89)	(0.04)	(0.39)
cation	−0.5	18	−10	−18	2	−32*
	(4.1)	(48)	(9)	(35)	(2)	(17)
n-Geest work	−32	−53	−24	200	25.6*	98
	(28)	(349)	(49)	(307)	(13.2)	(143)
gnancies	0.5		−2		−6.1*	
	(6.7)		(5)		(3.3)	
st housing	14	−37	−32	85	18	133
	(33)	(86)	(45)	(264)	(16)	(149)
w own bananas	−9	77*	1	388*	3	−91
	(7)	(44)	(59)	(220)	(4)	(129)
	0.41	0.37	0.57	0.24	0.44	0.31
atio	1.32	1.25	1.24	1.04	1.92	0.73

Carrying bananas from the field to loading point.
Wrapping banana stalks. This task is performed only by females.
Planting banana plants.
Digging drainage canals. This task is performed only by males.
* Significant at the .10 level (two-tailed test).
** Significant at the .05 level (two-tailed test).
*** Significant at the .01 level (two-tailed test).

Table D.7. Additive Model Regression Coefficients (and Standard Errors), Geest Workers, Mean Days Worked Per Week as Dependent Variable

Independent variable	Coefficients (and standard errors)	
	Males (N = 45) (1)	Females (N = 23) (2)
Constant	−3* (2)	1.2 (1.99)
Schistosoma		
Few eggs	.43 (.53)	.04 (.74)
Many eggs	1.12** (.53)	−.16 (.62)
Ascaris	−.41 (.44)	−.88 (.67)
Trichuris	.25 (.43)	.08 (.74)
Hookworm	−.15 (.45)	—
Strongyloides	—	−1.19* (.63)
Age	.27*** (.09)	.13 (.09)
Age squared	−.003*** (.001)	−.001 (.001)
Education	−.09 (.08)	−.02 (.07)
Non-Geest work	.69 (.51)	.12 (.71)
Pregnancies	—	−.00 (.02)
Geest housing	1.34** (.54)	−.13 (.65)
Grow own bananas	−1.00* (.55)	.22 (1.21)
R²	.47	.45
F ratio	2.82**	.45

Note: Dashes indicate insufficient observations.
  * Significant at the .10 level (two-tailed test).
 ** Significant at the .05 level (two-tailed test).
*** Significant at the .01 level (two-tailed test).

Clinical Symptoms

For the banana-plantation workers we have the results of clinical examinations to determine the presence or absence of physiological effects as indicated by (1) an enlarged liver, (2) enlarged spleen, (3) low hemoglobin count, or (4) such subjective symptoms as frequent abdominal or intestinal distress. The sample of persons for whom such information is available was not large enough to permit inclusion of these symptom variables in our agricultural productivity studies. Table D.8, however, compares the average daily earnings and the average number of days worked per week (over a six-month period) for a "healthy" group and for a "sick" group of workers. The former group was defined to include persons who (a) showed negative on all of two or more separate tests for the presence of schistosome eggs, and who (b) evidenced none of the four clinical symptoms listed above. The "sick" group was defined as persons who (a) showed positive evidence of schistosomiasis on one or more tests, and who (b) had at least two of the four clinical symptoms.

Table D.8. Mean Earnings Per Day and Days Worked Per Week for "Healthy" and "Sick" Geest Workers from Clinical Group

Variable	"Healthy" group	"Sick" group
Mean earnings per day (E.C. dollars)		
Males	$2.51 (N = 8)	$2.98 (N = 6)
Females	$1.74 (N = 9)	$1.94 (N = 13)
Mean days worked per week		
Males	4.47 (N = 8)	4.71 (N = 6)
Females	4.50 (N = 9)	4.30 (N = 13)

Clinical examinations were given to some three hundred fifty Geest workers, but Table D.8 includes data on only thirty-six of the workers, 10 percent of the total. The attrition was attributable to our definition of "healthy"—including only persons for whom at least two stool tests were done and who, in addition, had no clinical symptoms—and to our definition of "sick"—including only persons who, in addition to having a positive stool test, had two or more symptoms. The vast majority of workers who were examined clinically fit into neither of these "extreme" categories.

Because of sample-size problems we could not control for age and other productivity-related characteristics. Thus, great meaning should not be attributed to these data. What they show is that the "healthy" workers, both male and female, earned less, not more per day; the healthy males also worked fewer days per week, while the healthy females worked somewhat more than their sick counterparts. Although most of the differences are not statistically significant owing to the small number of observations (only the differential in earnings for males was significant; this was at the .05 level), they certainly provide scant evidence of debilitating effects of schistosomiasis infection.

It is also notable that the symptoms of severe schistosomiasis infection cannot be attributed specifically to that disease [143]. Our own evidence is thus consistent with medical knowledge suggesting that there are other sources of those symptoms, so that even if we had found adverse behavioral effects associated with presence of such symptoms, we would not be right in automatically attributing those effects to schistosomiasis. Table D.9 shows the frequencies of the various symptoms in a sample of thirty-two Geest workers who were infected with schistosomiasis and who had at least forty schistosome eggs per gram of stool, and in a sample of ap-

Table D.9. Association of Clinical Symptoms for Schistosomiasis with Stool-Specimen Diagnosis among Geest Workers

	Percentage of Geest workers having the stated symptom	
Symptom	Persons showing *S. mansoni* negative on two or more tests (N = 43)	Persons showing *S. mansoni* positive, with egg count of at least 40 eggs per gram (N = 32)
Enlarged spleen	4.7%	3.1%
Enlarged liver	9.3	9.4
"Low" hemoglobin count		
Less than 9 gram percent	9.3	15.6
Less than 12 gram percent	62.8	53.1
Abdominal/intestinal complaint	20.9	25.0

parently noninfected workers—those for whom no schistosome eggs were found in two or more independent stool tests. While there is always the possibility of false negatives even with two tests, it is nonetheless striking that no clear pattern of differential symptom frequency appears.

Disease and Urban-Labor Productivity

We hypothesized in the section above that if workers are being debilitated by schistosomiasis and other parasitic diseases, persons with these infections would earn less per week (hypothesis 1), be less productive per day worked (hypothesis 3), and be absent more (hypothesis 4). These expectations may be reasonable on the Geest plantation, where hard physical labor is involved, but may be inappropriate for more sedentary occupations. To test this possibility we used the data, described in chapter 5, on urban females working at paper-folding jobs for Dimensions, Ltd. Each of the three hypotheses was tested with the linear multiple regression approach used earlier. The disease-interaction approach was not utilized because of the large number of interaction variables for which there were only a few observations.

The results of our test of hypothesis 1, where the dependent variable is weekly salary, are given in column 5 of Table D.10. Columns 2–4 of Table D.10 show the test results of the hypothesis that workers infected with parasites are less productive while working than their "healthier" coworkers; the dependent variable is physical output on each of three separate jobs. The hypothesis that infected workers are absent more was tested by regressing the dependent variable, number of days worked as a percentage of potential work days (this was to adjust for the fact that some workers were hired later than others), on the independent variables enumerated above. The resulting estimates are in Table D.10, column 1.

Tables D.11 and D.12 summarize the findings with respect to our different measures of labor productivity. The remaining tables, D.13a–D.13c, D.14a, D.14b, D.15, are the zero order correlation matrices for the Geest plantation data and the Dimensions, Ltd., factory data.

Table D.10. Dimensions, Ltd, Regression Coefficients (and Standard Errors)

| Independent variable | Proportion of days worked (1) | Physical output per day[a] | | | Weekly salary (E.C. dollars) (5) |
		Job 1 (2)	Job 2 (3)	Job 3 (4)	
Constant	1.21	64.8	10.1	33.0**	14.04***
	(0.13)	(65.8)	(30.5)	(16.4)	(3.62)
Schistosoma	−0.004	−3.44	−1.28	−1.77	−0.025
	(0.012)	(6.13)	(2.85)	(1.31)	(0.338)
Hookworm	0.004	2.38	0.97	2.15**	0.227
	(0.010)	(4.81)	(2.31)	(1.06)	(0.265)
Ascaris	−0.002	−3.97	−2.52	−2.24*	−0.540
	(0.012)	(6.08)	(2.82)	(1.29)	(0.335)
Trichuris	−0.006	−0.81	−0.76	−1.63	−0.017
	(0.010)	(4.98)	(2.32)	(1.09)	(0.274)
Strongyloides	0.002	25.70	7.10	1.53	0.813
	(0.031)	(15.84)	(8.24)	(3.54)	(0.872)
Age	−.026**	5.96	2.27	−1.15	−0.23
	(.012)	(5.97)	(2.83)	(1.53)	(0.33)
Age squared	0.001	−0.157	−0.051	0.02	0.007
	(0.000)	(0.136)	(0.066)	(0.04)	(0.008)
Years of schooling	0.003	−49.9*	−3.8	−6.59	−1.43
	(0.050)	(25.2)	(10.4)	(4.74)	(1.38)
Marital status	−0.012	4.95	−0.10	0.13	0.018
	(0.015)	(7.48)	(4.41)	(1.92)	(0.412)
Number of dependents	−0.012**	2.30	0.67	0.25	−0.060
	(0.006)	(2.95)	(1.50)	(0.69)	(0.162)
Urban vs. other residence	−0.035**	19.00**	1.37	1.95	−0.010
	(0.016)	(7.87)	(3.68)	(1.73)	(0.433)
Semi-urban vs. other residence	−0.022	19.21**	3.20	0.93	−0.166
	(0.017)	(8.42)	(3.90)	(1.86)	(0.464)
R^2	0.148	0.103	0.061	0.175	0.116
F ratio	1.47	0.98	0.40	1.23	1.11

Note: Sample sizes (number of workers) for each of the dependent variables are as follows: columns 1, 2, 5: N = 114; column 3: N = 86; column 4: N = 82.

[a] The three jobs listed below are basically all the same type of work—folding and pasting advertising material. The jobs are distinguished because they represent different orders for different firms; consequently, there are likely to be quantitative and qualitative differences in the folding and pasting operations.

* Significant at the .10 level.
** Significant at the .05 level.
*** Significant at the .01 level.

Table D.11 (title partially illegible)

Geest workers

Variable	Earnings per week M (1)	F (2)	M (3)	F (4)	Task days worked as % of total days worked M (5)	F (6)	Earnings per day worked M (7)	F (8)	Earnings per day — Task 1[a] M (9)	F (10)	Task 2[b] F (11)	Task 3[c] M (12)	F (13)	Task 4[d] M (14)	Days worked per week M (15)	F (16)
Schistosoma	0	0	0	0	0	0	−	0	0	0	0	0	+	0	+	0
Ascaris	0	0	0	0	0	0	0	0	−	−	0	−	0	0	0	0
Trichuris	0	0	0	0	0	0	0	0	0	+	0	0	0	0	0	0
Hookworm	0	0	0	1	0	1	0	1	0	0	0	0	0	0	0	1
Strongyloides	0	0	1	−	1	0	1	−	0	0	0	0	0	0	1	−

Dimensions, Ltd., workers

Variable	Physical output per day[e] Job 1 (17)	Job 2 (18)	Job 3 (19)	% of days worked (20)	Earnings per week (21)	Summary number of +'s (22)	−'s (23)	0's (24)	Total test performance (25)
Schistosoma	0	0	0	0	0	2	1	18	21
Ascaris	0	0	−	0	0	0	4	17	21
Trichuris	0	0	0	0	0	1	0	20	21
Hookworm	0	0	+	0	0	1	0	16	17
Strongyloides	0	0	0	0	0	0	3	14	17
Total						4	8	85	97

Source: Tables D.3–D.7, D.10. Note: + = significant at .10 level or better, and positive; − = significant at .10 level or better, and negative; 0 = not significantly different from zero; 1 = insufficient observations.

a Carrying bananas from the field to loading point.
b Wrapping banana stalks. This task is performed only by females.
c Planting banana plants.
d Digging drainage canals. This task is performed only by males.
e See Table D.10, note a.

Table D.12. Summary of Findings, Nondisease Variables

	Geest workers												
	Earnings per week						Task days worked as % of total days worked		Earnings per days worked		Earnings p[er] Task 1[a]		Task 2[b]
Variable	M (1)	F (2)	M (3)	F (4)	M (5)	F (6)	M (7)	F (8)	M (9)	F (10)	M (11)	F (12)	F (13)
Age	0	0	0	0	0	+	0	0	0	+	0	0	0
Age squared	0	0	0	0	0	−	0	0	0	−	0	0	0
Yrs. of school	0	0	0	0	0	0	0	0	0	0	0	0	0
Non-Geest work	0	0	0	0	0	0	0	0	−	0	0	0	0
No. of preg.		0		0		0		0		0			0
Geest housing	0	0	0	0	0	0	0	0	0	0	0	0	0
Grow own bananas	0	0	0	0	0	0	0	0	0	0	+	0	0
Martial status													
No. of dependents													
Urban vs. other residence													
Semi-urban vs. other residence													
Total													

Source: Tables D.2–D.7, D.10.

Note: + = significant, at .10 level or better, and positive; − = significant, at .10 level or better, and negative; 0 = not significantly different from zero.

  a Carrying bananas from the field to loading point.

  b Wrapping banana stalks. This task is performed only by females.

  c Planting banana plants.

  d Digging drainage canals. This task is performed only by males.

  e See Table D.10, note a.

						Dimensions, Ltd., workers							
ay worked at		Task 4d	Days worked per week		Physical output per day			% of days	Earnings per week	Summary no. of			Total test performance
Task 3c								worked					
M	F	M	M	F	Job 1	Job 2	Job 3			+'s	−'s	0's	
(14)	(15)	(16)	(17)	(18)	(19)	(20)	(21)	(22)	(23)	(24)	(25)	(26)	(27)
0	0	0	+	0	0	0	0	−	0	3	1	19	23
0	0	0	−	0	0	0	0	0	0	0	3	20	23
0	0	−	0	0	−	0	0	0	0	0	2	21	23
0	+	0	0	0						1	1	16	18
		−		0						0	1	8	9
0	0	0	+	0						1	0	17	18
+	0	0	−	0						2	1	15	18
					0	0	0	0	0	0	0	5	5
					0	0	0	−	0	0	1	4	5
					+	0	0	−	0	1	1	33	35
					+	0	0	0	0	1	0	4	5
										9	11	162	182

Table D.13a. Geest Worker Correlation Matrix—Males

	Age (2)	Schistosoma (3)	Hookworm (4)	Ascaris (5)	Trichuris (6)	Strongyloides (7)	Education (8)	Non-Geest work (9)	Liver & spleen (10)	Hemoglobin (11)	Geest housing (13)	Grow bananas (14)	Migration (15)	Days worked per week (16)	Earnings per week (17)
Age (2)	1.000	-0.051	0.049	0.199	-0.264	0.218	-0.190	-0.155	-0.092	-0.328	0.138	-0.154	-0.165	0.220	0.249
Schistosoma (3)		1.000	0.047	-0.105	0.146	0.107	-0.313	0.244	0.207	-0.121	0.170	0.207	0.133	-0.011	-0.038
Hookworm (4)			1.000	-0.057	0.207	0.153	-0.017	-0.153	0.112	-0.019	0.141	-0.058	-0.168	0.209	-0.027
Ascaris (5)				1.000	-0.021	-0.039	-0.285	-0.031	-0.089	-0.056	0.053	-0.005	0.094	-0.138	-0.050
Trichuris (6)					1.000	-0.017	0.022	0.017	0.047	0.179	-0.032	0.211	0.114	-0.186	-0.191
Strongyloides (7)						1.000	0.083	-0.088	0.004	-0.142	0.529	-0.087	-0.044	0.231	0.078
Education (8)							1.000	-0.052	-0.141	-0.006	0.049	0.049	-0.043	0.163	-0.174
Non-Geest work (9)								1.000	0.087	-0.083	-0.134	0.269	0.172	0.009	0.033
Liver & spleen (10)									1.000	0.189	0.319	0.021	0.027	-0.155	-0.008
Hemoglobin (11)										1.000	0.042	0.279	0.053	-0.172	-0.184
Geest housing (13)											1.000	0.035	0.107	0.188	0.099
Grow bananas (14)												1.000	0.334	-0.017	-0.152
Migration (15)													1.000	-0.085	0.008
Days worked per week (16)														1.000	0.193
Earnings per week (17)															1.000

Table D.13b. Geest Worker Correlation Matrix—Males

	Age squared (22)	% worked on task (23)	Earnings per day (24)	H, A (36)	Sc, H (48)	Sc, H, St, T (49)	Sc, H, T (50)	Sc, H, A (52)	Sc, H, A, T (54)	Sc, H, A, T, St (55)	Task earnings per day (56)	Days worked earnings per day (57)		
Age	0.984	-0.153	0.086	-0.096	-0.133	0.133	-0.263	0.275	-0.167	0.055	-0.191	0.131	Age	2
Schistosoma	-0.043	0.259	-0.066	-0.608	0.160	0.133	0.146	0.218	0.207	0.133	0.201	-0.095	Schistosoma	3
Hookworm	0.068	0.049	-0.195	0.072	0.086	0.072	0.079	0.118	0.112	0.072	0.100	-0.178	Hookworm	4
Ascaris	0.203	-0.066	0.014	0.212	-0.047	-0.380	-0.420	0.349	0.331	0.212	-0.104	0.038	Ascaris	5
Trichuris	-0.260	0.144	0.014	-0.233	-0.281	-0.233	0.382	-0.384	0.539	0.346	0.299	-0.012	Trichuris	6
Strongyloides	0.225	0.112	-0.186	-0.172	-0.207	0.469	-0.190	-0.283	-0.269	0.469	0.204	-0.191	Strongyloides	7
Education	-0.168	-0.245	-0.248	0.100	0.031	-0.043	0.071	-0.274	-0.115	-0.114	-0.069	-0.214	Education	8
Non-Geest work	-0.222	0.336	-0.076	-0.084	0.097	-0.084	-0.046	0.020	0.087	-0.084	0.324	-0.122	Non-Geest work	9
Liver & spleen	-0.056	-0.015	0.060	-0.126	0.112	0.027	0.002	0.108	0.021	0.027	-0.044	0.065	Liver & spleen	10
Hemoglobin	-0.353	0.096	-0.037	0.053	-0.002	-0.199	0.197	-0.138	0.011	-0.073	0.147	-0.073	Hemoglobin	11
Geest housing	0.133	-0.102	-0.073	-0.159	-0.077	0.241	-0.176	-0.079	-0.059	0.241	0.002	-0.058	Geest housing	13
Grow bananas	-0.176	0.285	-0.088	-0.126	-0.020	-0.126	0.143	-0.102	0.239	-0.126	0.344	-0.172	Grow bananas	14
Migration	-0.186	-0.006	0.082	-0.081	0.089	-0.081	-0.089	-0.133	0.181	0.135	0.103	0.005	Migration	15
Days worked per week	0.164	-0.074	-0.571	-0.028	0.189	0.193	-0.204	-0.081	-0.049	0.087	-0.023	-0.547	Days worked per week	16
Earnings per week	0.220	-0.124	0.609	0.065	0.100	0.072	-0.090	0.058	-0.218	0.098	-0.081	0.591	Earnings per week	17

Note: A = Ascaris, H = Hookworm, Sc = Schistosoma, St = Strongyloides, T = Trichuris.

Table D.13c. Geest Worker Correlation Matrix—Males

	Age squared (22)	% worked on task (23)	Earnings per day (24)	H, A (36)	Sc, H (48)	Sc, H, St, T (49)	Sc, H, T (50)	Sc, H, A (52)	Sc, H, A, T (54)	Sc, H, A, T, St (55)	Task earnings per day (56)	Days worked earnings per day (57)	
Age squared	1.000	−0.199	0.097	−0.116	−0.122	0.125	−0.264	0.275	−0.155	0.041	−0.239	0.147	22
% worked on task		1.000	−0.110	−0.125	−0.039	−0.102	0.203	0.058	−0.099	0.106	0.759	−0.208	23
Earnings per day			1.000	0.040	−0.032	−0.076	0.130	0.062	−0.119	−0.038	−0.119	0.972	24
H, A				1.000	−0.097	−0.081	−0.089	−0.133	−0.126	−0.081	−0.092	0.051	36
Sc, H					1.000	−0.097	−0.107	−0.160	−0.151	−0.097	−0.087	−0.064	48
Sc, H, St, T						1.000	−0.089	−0.133	−0.126	−0.081	−0.061	−0.061	49
Sc, H, T							1.000	−0.146	−0.139	−0.089	0.133	0.093	50
Sc, H, A								1.000	−0.207	−0.133	−0.065	0.091	52
Sc, H, A, T									1.000	−0.126	−0.030	−0.094	54
Sc, H, A, T, St										1.000	0.261	−0.085	55
Task earnings per day											1.000	−0.193	56
Days worked earnings per day												1.000	57

Note: A = *Ascaris*, H = Hookworm, Sc = *Schistosoma*, St = *Strongyloides*, T = *Trichuris*.

Table D.14a. Geest Worker Correlation Matrix—Females

	Age (2)	*Schistosoma* (3)	Hookworm (4)	*Ascaris* (5)	*Trichuris* (6)	*Strongyloides* (7)	Education (8)	Non-Geest work (9)	Liver and spleen (10)	Hemoglobin (11)	Pregnancies (12)	Geest housing (13)	Grow bananas (14)	Migration (15)	Days worked per week (16)	Earnings per week (17)
Age (2)	1.000	-0.334	-0.047	-0.350	-0.250	0.107	-0.259	-0.122	0.104	0.135	0.555	0.036	0.222	0.145	0.263	0.128
Schistosoma (3)		1.000	0.043	0.340	0.263	0.069	0.035	0.119	0.000	-0.133	-0.216	0.253	-0.216	-0.066	-0.211	-0.016
Hookworm (4)			1.000	0.070	-0.010	-0.059	-0.080	0.142	0.101	-0.091	-0.017	-0.054	-0.173	0.056	-0.098	0.014
Ascaris (5)				1.000	0.369	-0.189	0.088	0.177	0.210	-0.039	-0.160	0.189	0.020	0.117	-0.168	-0.104
Trichuris (6)					1.000	-0.066	-0.022	0.057	-0.169	0.051	-0.307	0.139	-0.016	0.157	-0.222	-0.137
Strongyloides (7)						1.000	-0.062	-0.046	0.033	-0.015	-0.011	-0.162	-0.126	-0.073	0.185	0.136
Education (8)							1.000	0.138	-0.066	0.043	-0.231	-0.124	-0.002	-0.099	0.032	0.009
Non-Geest work (9)								1.000	-0.067	-0.147	-0.048	-0.234	-0.040	0.212	-0.036	0.062
Liver & spleen (10)									1.000	0.050	-0.079	0.131	-0.082	-0.062	0.014	-0.056
Hemoglobin (11)										1.000	0.040	0.157	-0.008	-0.112	0.158	0.123
Pregnancies (12)											1.000	-0.117	0.045	0.145	0.220	0.208
Geest housing (13)												1.000	-0.042	-0.126	-0.037	-0.044
Grow bananas (14)													1.000	0.314	0.252	0.114
Migration (15)														1.000	0.134	0.134
Days worked per week (16)															1.000	0.902
Earnings per week (17)																1.000

Table D. 14b. Geest Worker Correlation Matrix—Females

	Age squared (22)	Percent worked on task (23)	Earnings per day (24)	H (32)	H, A, T (38)	Sc, H, A (52)	Sc, H, A, T (54)	Task earnings per day (56)	Days worked earnings per day (57)	
Age	0.980	-0.223	-0.076	0.124	-0.080	0.042	-0.252	-0.234	0.032	2
Sc	-0.345	0.160	0.356	-0.471	-0.471	0.236	0.500	0.191	0.292	3
H	-0.050	0.049	0.129	0.101	0.101	0.101	0.213	0.163	0.119	4
A	-0.338	0.131	-0.115	-0.530	0.210	0.210	0.445	0.044	-0.206	5
T	-0.236	0.148	0.052	-0.394	0.282	-0.394	0.598	0.068	-0.083	6
St	0.137	-0.181	-0.044	-0.131	-0.131	-0.131	-0.277	-0.108	0.086	7
Education	-0.231	-0.067	-0.119	-0.177	0.247	0.210	-0.070	0.043	-0.061	8
Non-Geest worker	-0.097	0.192	0.147	0.045	0.045	0.045	0.095	0.034	0.091	9
Liver & spleen	0.059	-0.259	-0.206	-0.111	0.074	0.259	-0.118	-0.374	-0.068	10
Hemoglobin	0.189	-0.060	0.059	0.050	0.050	-0.075	0.053	0.025	0.114	11
Pregnancies	0.539	0.067	0.065	0.219	-0.100	0.240	-0.243	0.080	0.043	12
Geest housing	0.036	-0.104	0.063	-0.227	-0.107	0.012	0.279	0.004	0.083	13
Grow bananas	0.195	-0.148	-0.176	-0.082	0.117	-0.107	-0.021	-0.098	-0.096	14
Migration	0.128	0.030	0.007	-0.062	0.248	-0.062	0.066	-0.072	0.004	15
Days worked per week	0.235	0.174	-0.029	0.017	-0.033	0.081	-0.212	0.229	-0.176	16
Earnings per week	0.083	0.466	0.338	-0.026	-0.076	0.111	-0.117	0.432	0.039	17
Age squared	1.000	-0.267	-0.123	0.129	-0.075	-0.019	-0.231	-0.272	0.012	22
% worked on task		1.000	0.522	0.003	-0.058	0.032	0.204	0.541	-0.091	23
Earnings per day			1.000	-0.067	-0.170	0.017	0.049	0.371	0.779	24
H				1.000	-0.111	-0.111	-0.236	0.115	-0.062	32
H, A, T					1.000	-0.111	-0.236	-0.032	-0.147	38
Sc, H, A						1.000		-0.021	0.043	52
Sc, H, A, T							1.000	0.056	-0.120	54
Task earnings per day								1.000	0.023	56
Days worked earnings per day									1.000	57

Note: A = *Ascaris*, H = Hookworm, Sc = *Schistosoma*, T = *Trichuris*.

162

Table D.15. Dimensions, Ltd., Correlation Matrix

	Age (1)	Education (2)	Married (3)	No. of live births (4)	No. of still-births (5)	Depend-ents (6)	Urban (7)	Semi-urban (8)	Schisto-soma (9)	Hook-worm (10)	Ascaris (11)	Trichuris (12)	Strongy-loides (13)	Salary (14)	Days worked (15)	% of days worked (16)	Average output (24)	
Age	1.000	0.105	0.628	0.738	0.452	0.740	0.154	-0.074	-0.041	-0.054	-0.153	-0.175	0.285	0.283	0.225	-0.046	0.113	1
Education		1.000	0.041	0.063	0.043	0.072	0.120	0.074	0.055	-0.109	0.051	-0.112	0.017	-0.128	0.066	-0.085	-0.014	2
Married			1.000	0.566	0.327	0.577	-0.074	0.182	-0.109	0.108	-0.002	-0.091	0.172	0.250	-0.001	-0.174	0.091	3
Live births				1.000	0.438	0.964	0.115	-0.027	-0.105	-0.129	-0.076	-0.193	0.299	0.177	0.073	-0.144	0.071	4
Stillbirths					1.000	0.512	0.092	-0.104	-0.007	-0.181	-0.120	-0.172	0.292	0.025	-0.044	-0.080	0.026	5
Dependents						1.000	0.146	-0.042	-0.137	-0.125	-0.078	-0.212	0.307	0.191	0.070	-0.180	0.124	6
Urban							1.000	-0.764	0.175	-0.080	0.070	0.085	-0.016	0.015	-0.134	-0.276	-0.073	7
Semi-urban								1.000	-0.048	0.106	-0.073	-0.173	-0.106	-0.039	-0.016	0.130	0.109	8
Schistosoma									1.000	-0.221	0.051	-0.210	-0.078	0.044	-0.096	-0.006	-0.063	9
Hookworm										1.000	0.183	0.287	0.002	0.004	0.059	0.064	0.038	10
Ascaris											1.000	0.195	-0.073	-0.212	-0.190	-0.075	-0.132	11
Trichuris												1.000	0.005	-0.063	-0.143	-0.013	-0.076	12
Strongyloides													1.000	0.223	0.164	0.106	0.097	13
Salary														1.000	0.629	0.256	0.526	14
Days worked															1.000	0.369	0.464	15
% of days worked																1.000	0.255	16
Average output																	1.000	24

Appendix E

SUPPLEMENTARY TABLES

Table E.1. Summary of Coefficient Signs for Disease Tests

Parasite	Geest[a]			Dimensions, Ltd.[b]			Geest and Dimensions, Ltd.		
	P (1)	U (2)	S.L. (3)	P (4)	U (5)	S.L. (6)	P (7)	U (8)	S.L. (9)
Schistosoma	13	11		5	0	*	18	11	
Ascaris	13	3	**	5	0	*	18	3	***
Trichuris	7	9		5	0	*	12	9	
Hookworm	8	4		0	5	*	8	9	
Strongyloides	9	3		0	5	*	9	8	
All parasites	50	30		15	10		65	40	**

Note: The results of all interaction model tests are excluded. P = predicted sign, U = unpredicted sign, and S.L. = significance level (two-tailed test).

[a] From Tables D.3–D.7.

[b] From Table D.10.

[c] From Table B.3.

[d] From Table B.5. Only the linear formulation was included to prevent double-counting of nonindependent data.

[e] From Tables C.7, C.10–C.13.

* = .10 significance level.

** = .05 significance level.

*** = .01 significance level.

Birth[c]			Death[d]			Education[e]			All		
P	U	S.L.	P	U	S.L.	P	U	S.L.	P	U	S.L.
(10)	(11)	(12)	(13)	(14)	(15)	(16)	(17)	(18)	(19)	(20)	(21)
1	1		0	1		8	3		27	16	
0	2		0	0		5	2		23	7	***
2	0		0	1		2	5		16	15	
1	1		1	0		3	4		13	14	
2	0		0	1		1	2		12	11	
6	4		1	3		19	16		91	63	**

Table E.2. Recent World-Wide Surveys of Prevalence Rates for Schistosomiasis (*S. mansoni*)

Country	Area	Year	Population	Prevalence
Brazil	Sao Paulo State	1957	2,611 persons of all ages	0.8%
			Of the above number, 1,396 were schoolchildren	1.1
Congo, Rep. Dem.	Ituri Forest	1963	232 Pygmies of all ages	7
Nigeria	Ibadan, Moor Plantation	1960	100 employees of 15–48 years, selected at random	8
Brazil	Gameleira, Pernambuco State	1959	148 (44%) of the children from 6 mos. to 3 years	8.8
Nigeria	Daiya (village)	1963	128 of local population	10
Uganda	Nile Province	1950–1955	7,064 persons over 5 years	13
Surinam		1956–1957	10,356 from a household survey	13
Nigeria	Yo	1963	162 irrigation project staff	15
Madagascar	Ambositra, Fianarantsoa Province	1959	566 adults from 21 hamlets	29
			381 children from 4 schools	18
St. Lucia	*Soufriere*	*1960*	*229 children, 4–14 years*	*33*
St. Lucia	*Cul-de-Sac Valley*	*1965*	*640 children, 4–14 years*	*46*
Brazil	Utinga, Alagoas State	1952–1953	1,636 males of all ages	47
			1,763 females of all ages	45
Ethiopia	Adwa, Tigre Province	1964	Stratified sample of the town	
			297 males	65
			162 females	56
Brazil	Vicosa Municipality, Alagoas State	1953–1956	41 persons of Camboim II	63
			114 persons of Nova Ouro	53
			217 persons of Rio Branco	68
Ethiopia	Harar, Harar Province	1961–1962	152 boys from Moslem school, average age 13 years	71

Source: This table includes all surveys listed in a W.H.O. literature review for the period 1959–1968, which tested for infection with the *S. mansoni* species alone [103].

Appendix F

ANALYSIS OF
DATA REPRESENTATIVENESS

Introduction

Since our several studies do not encompass the entire St. Lucian population, but rather deal with samples of certain selected subgroups or classes of the total population, we need to consider whether there might be any health biases in these studies. Specifically, we are concerned whether, because of our own conscious selection of population subgroups or because of the nature of our sampling procedures within those groups, we might have selectively studied persons with lower infection levels than the overall St. Lucian population.[1]

This appendix considers each of the bodies of data we used and discusses the representativeness of those samples to the entire population of such people—agricultural workers or students, for example. Throughout, we will be concerned primarily with the question of whether our samples are systematically biased toward persons who are infected less by parasites and who may be less severely affected by the parasites—that is, may be less "sick" in a behavioral sense.

---

1. "Infection level," here, refers both to prevalence and to intensity. Though prevalence and intensity are separate and distinct measures of infection, we will utilize—in the absence of better measures of comparative intensity—the argument that groups of persons with relatively high infection *prevalence* levels are likely to also have relatively high infection *intensity* levels.

Cul-de-Sac Valley and Roseau Valley
Household Surveys

ISLAND-WIDE REPRESENTATIVENESS

A key question with regard to our household surveys in Cul-de-Sac Valley and Roseau Valley is whether the populations of these two rural valleys are representative of the rural population of St. Lucia. Our decision to conduct household surveys in Cul-de-Sac and Roseau was directed by the prior decision of the Research and Control Department schistosomiasis-research team to conduct parasitological surveys in these valleys. The Research and Control Department team selected these two valleys, plus Riche Fond Valley,[2] because of their apparent suitability for later study of the comparative effectiveness of alternative schistosomiasis-control measures.[3] Though large-scale household parasitological surveys have been conducted only in these valleys, much more limited surveys, conducted in other areas of the island, suggest that the valleys included in our study are not subaverage in terms of parasite infection levels.

Cul-de-Sac and Roseau residents include wage-laborers, private banana growers—producing bananas on their own small plots of land—and families subsisting through the production of ground provisions. These latter two groups are probably typical of rural persons in other parts of the small—twenty-seven miles, greatest length; fourteen miles, greatest breadth —island. These two valleys are atypical, however, in the dominance of the large banana plantations, owned by the firm Geest Industries. Some observers feel that these foreign-owned plantations evoke memories of slavery. The plantation laborers—some 25 percent of the adult population of the valleys—generally own no land of their own, and are said to be resentfully conscious of a lack of independence. These factors may well be of socio-cultural significance, but we do not find them likely to lead to below-average levels of parasitic infection.[4]

REPRESENTATIVENESS OF PERSONS SURVEYED

A second question is whether our samples within the Cul-de-Sac and Roseau valleys are representative of the entire population of these valleys. The Research and Control Department's parasitological survey sought

2. We began, but did not complete, a household survey in Riche Fond because only limited transportation facilities were available to us.

3. No control measures had yet been implemented at the time our studies were completed.

4. The plantations, by bringing large numbers of workers together, might increase the transmission potentiality of some parasites. No special precautionary measures for reducing transmission were practiced on the plantations.

to include all households within the respective valley watersheds. We, in turn, sought to apply our economic survey to all households from which stool specimens were obtained on the parasitological survey, though (as described below) we also visited many households from which parasitological data were not obtained.

Because the parasitological survey in Cul-de-Sac was already underway when we began operations in St. Lucia, our economic survey in Cul-de-Sac followed the parasitological survey there by several months. In Roseau, however, the parasitological and economic surveys were conducted simultaneously. The parasitological survey team (operating alone in Cul-de-Sac and with the economic survey interviewer in Roseau) found "closed" households in each valley, for which no occupant was at home when the team visited the household. In consequence, no stool-specimen tins were distributed to these households. For the "open" households, to all members of which stool-specimen tins were distributed, we distinguish between the "respondents," who returned stools, and the nonrespondents, who did not.

Although the parasitological survey team made only one attempt to survey a household, our economic survey interviewer made repeat visits in one of the valleys, Cul-de-Sac, in an attempt to obtain coverage of all persons included in the parasitological survey sample. In addition, our Cul-de-Sac interviewer surveyed households that were originally listed as "closed" by the parasitological survey team. As a result, we have descriptive data on a group of Cul-de-Sac persons who had been excluded from the parasite-test sample. We can, therefore, compare these persons with the group for whom we obtained parasite information, to determine whether our parasite-test sample was markedly different from the group of persons for which no parasite data were obtained. In Roseau Valley, where the parasitological and economic surveys were conducted simultaneously, the merged teams made only one visit to each household. Thus, no information is available on characteristics of the nonsurveyed population of that valley.

The response rates to the parasitological and economic surveys, in Cul-de-Sac Valley and Roseau Valley, are summarized in Table F.1. We note, for example, that the parasitological survey found 80.2 percent of Cul-de-Sac houses "open," and that stool specimens were obtained from 65.8 percent of the occupants of these houses.

Tables F.2, F.4, F.6, and F.7 compare the age, sex, educational, and occupational distributions for Cul-de-Sac persons from whom parasitological data were and were not obtained—both those who were missed because no one was home at the time of the parasitological survey team visit, and those who received, but did not return, a stool-specimen container. Tables F.3 and F.5, which present the age and sex parasite-preva-

Table F.1. Cul-de-Sac and Roseau Valley Household Surveys Response Rates, 1967–1968

Variable	Cul-de-Sac Valley	Roseau Valley
Total houses in valley	1,060	790
Percentage of total houses open to parasitological survey	80.2	78.2
Percentage of total houses open to economic survey	92.7[a]	74.4[b]
Persons surveyed by parasitological team	4,326	3,190
Percentage of persons on parasitological survey returning stool specimens	65.8	74.2
Persons surveyed by economic team	4,808	2,996

[a] Some of the 7.3 percent of Cul-de-Sac houses not surveyed were not occupied.

[b] Though the economic and parasitological surveys were conducted simultaneously in Roseau Valley, on two nonconsecutive occasions the parasitological survey was conducted in the absence of the economic survey interviewer, who was ill. The houses covered by the parasitological survey team during these two days are excluded from the economic survey.

Table F.2. Age Distribution of Cul-de-Sac Valley Persons for Whom Parasitological Data Were and Were Not Available, 1967–1968

Age[a]	Persons for whom parasito-logical data were available[b]	Persons for whom no parasitological data were available		
		Total[c]	Non-respondents[d]	Persons not initially sampled[e]
under 2 years	3.7%	5.4%	5.0%	6.3%
2–5	16.3	18.2	18.3	17.8
6–9	14.2	12.0	12.5	10.5
10–14	14.7	10.0	10.2	9.5
15–19	9.5	9.0	9.5	7.5
20–29	10.5	13.6	13.4	14.1
30–44	14.8	15.3	14.2	18.7
45–59	9.9	11.2	11.7	9.7
60+	6.5	5.4	5.2	5.8
Total	100.1%[f]	100.1%[f]	100%	99.9%[f]

[a] In a few instances—less than .5 percent of the total survey population—the interviewer recorded a question mark for "age." These have been deleted from the table.

[b] 2,342 persons interviewed on the economic survey who also returned stool specimens on the parasitological survey.

[c] 1,640 nonrespondents plus persons not initially sampled.

[d] 1,229 persons interviewed on the economic survey who, though provided with stool-specimen containers by the parasitological survey, did not return specimens.

[e] 411 persons from houses found "closed" by the parasitological survey, but interviewed during the economic survey.

[f] Age groups do not add to 100.0 percent due to rounding.

Table F.3. Cul-de-Sac Valley Parasitological Survey: Age-Prevalence Structure, 1967

| Age | Persons tested | | | Persons found to have each parasite | | | |
		Schisto-soma	Hook-worm	Ascaris	Trichuris	Strongy-loides	All parasite average[a]
under 2 years	180	3.3%	7.2%	40.0%	25.6%	2.8%	15.8%
2–5	481	23.7	31.4	53.0	62.6	6.9	35.5
6–9	398	43.0	42.5	55.5	68.1	10.3	43.9
10–14	397	57.7	51.4	55.2	67.8	12.6	48.9
15–19	252	58.3	60.7	48.8	61.5	14.3	48.7
20–24	146	46.6	62.3	41.1	45.9	17.1	42.6
25–29	139	38.9	66.2	44.6	48.2	15.8	42.7
30–44	429	32.4	69.9	40.1	51.3	20.3	42.8
45–59	275	32.0	74.6	34.2	45.8	23.3	42.0
60+	168	32.1	73.2	33.3	51.2	20.2	42.0

[a] The average prevalence of all five parasites in the age group.

lence structures, respectively, of the parasitological survey population, are auxiliary to the interpretation of Tables F.2 and F.4.

Table F.2 reveals that the parasite-tested group was somewhat biased in favor of the 6–19 years age range. Because the prevalence of each of the parasite infections is highly age-specific (Table F.3),[5] this age struc-

Table F.4. Sex Distribution of Cul-de-Sac Valley Persons for Whom Parasitological Data Were and Were Not Available, 1967–1968

| Sex distribution | Persons for whom parasito-logical data were available[a] | Persons for whom no parasitological data were available | | |
		Total[b]	Non-respondents[c]	Persons not initially sampled[d]
Male	46.9%	50.6%	50.2%	52.0%
Female	53.1	49.4	49.8	48.0
Total	100%	100%	100%	100%

[a] 2,342 persons interviewed on the economic survey who also returned stool specimens on the parasitological survey.

[b] 1,640 nonrespondents plus persons not initially sampled.

[c] 1,229 persons interviewed on the economic survey who, though provided with stool-specimen containers by the parasitological survey, did not return specimens.

[d] 411 persons from houses found "closed" by the parasitological survey, but interviewed during the economic survey.

5. All five parasites, individually as well as the five-parasite infection average, have highly significant (.01 level) age specificity.

Table F.5. Cul-de-Sac Valley Parasitological Survey: Sex-Prevalence Rates, 1967

Sex	Persons tested	Persons found to have each parasite					
		Schisto-soma*	Hook-worm***	Ascaris	Trichuris	Strongy-loides***	All parasite average[a]
Males (2+ years)	1,246	37.9%	60.4%	46.6%	57.5%	17.3%	43.9%
Females (2+ years)	1,439	41.1	51.2	47.3	58.7	12.3	42.1

[a] The average prevalence of all five parasites in the grouping.
* The difference in prevalence rates for males and females is significant at the .10 level.
*** The difference in prevalence rates for males and females is significant at the .01 level.

ture bias will contribute to the finding that our parasite-tested group has *higher* overall prevalences of *Schistosoma, Ascaris,* and *Trichuris* and lower overall prevalences of hookworm and *Strongyloides* than does the population as a whole. In general, however, it appears from Table F.2 that the age distribution of the sample for whom we obtained parasite

Table F.6. Educational Distribution of Cul-de-Sac Valley Persons for Whom Parasitological Data Were and Were Not Available, 1967–1968

Education class	Persons for whom parasito-logical data were available[a]	Persons for whom no parasitological data were available		
		Total[b]	Non-respondents[c]	Persons not initially sampled[d]
0	15.0%	23.0%	20.6%	30.2%
Pre-primary	21.6	22.1	23.5	18.0
Early primary (Standards 1–3)	25.7	23.6	24.4	21.2
Late primary (Standards 4–6)	35.5	30.1	30.2	29.7
Secondary (Forms 1+)	2.1	1.2	1.4	0.9
Total	99.9%[e]	100%	100.1%[e]	100%

Note: In a number of instances (21 percent of total population surveyed) a question mark appeared in the education column on the economic survey. These are deleted from the data in this table. Also deleted are "dash" entries which were descriptive of preschool aged children (essentially under age six).

[a] 1,416 persons interviewed on the economic survey who also returned stool specimens on the parasitological survey.

[b] 891 nonrespondents plus persons not initially sampled.

[c] 669 persons interviewed on the economic survey who, though provided with stool-specimen containers by the parasitological survey, did not return specimens.

[d] 222 persons from houses found "closed" by the parasitological survey, but interviewed during the economic survey.

[e] Classes do not add to 100.0 percent due to rounding.

data is not markedly unlike the age distribution of the population for whom such data were not obtained.

Table F.4 shows the sex distributions of the tested and nontested groups. It reveals that our sample has a somewhat higher percentage of females than does the nontested population—53.1 percent vs. 49.4 percent. This is relevant since the prevalence rates of several of the parasitic infections are highly sex-specific. As Table F.5 shows, the difference in prevalence rates between males and females in Cul-de-Sac is statistically significant for *Schistosoma* (.10 level), hookworm (.01 level), and *Strongyloides* (.01 level). The sex-prevalence differences for *Ascaris, Trichuris,* and for the five-parasite average infection level, however, are not significant at the .10 level. Consequently, we estimate that the pro-female bias of the tested group contributes to a somewhat higher overall prevalence of *Schistosoma* and to somewhat lower overall prevalences of hookworm and *Strongyloides* in our sample, compared to the group for whom parasite data were not obtained. Overall, there is little reason to believe that the sampled group is distorted in favor of uninfected ("healthier") persons.

Education is another dimension, in addition to age and sex, by which we can compare the sampled and nonsampled groups. The comparative

Table F.7. Occupational Distribution of Cul-de-Sac Valley Persons for Whom Parasitological Data Were and Were Not Available (Ages 15–65), 1967–1968

| Occupational class | Persons for whom parasito-logical data were available[a] | Persons for whom no parasitological data were available | | |
		Total[b]	Non-respondents[c]	Persons not initially sampled[d]
Geest banana plantation	12.0%	15.1%	12.5%	22.4%
Private banana grower	8.2	7.3	7.5	6.8
Laborer	30.8	33.3	34.9	29.1
Other work	23.5	21.4	22.4	18.6
Not employed	25.5	22.9	22.8	23.2
Total	100%	100%	100.1%[e]	100.1%[e]

[a] 1,144 persons interviewed on the economic survey who also returned stool specimens on the parasitological survey.

[b] 894 nonrespondents plus persons not initially sampled.

[c] 657 persons interviewed on the economic survey who, though provided with stool-specimen containers by the parasitological survey, did not return specimens.

[d] 237 persons from houses found "closed" by the parasitological survey, but interviewed during the economic survey.

[e] Classes do not add to 100.0 percent due to rounding.

educational-status distribution (Table F.6) reveals that persons with more education tended to be tested in greater proportion than those of lesser education. It is a plausible hypothesis that the better educated might tend to be more successful than the lesser educated in avoiding serious infections, but this remains to be tested.

Finally, we can compare the sampled and nonsampled groups in terms of their occupational distributions (Table F.7). It is especially notable that the unemployed—those whom one might consider most likely to be seriously affected by their parasite infections—were actually *over*-represented in our tested group; they constituted 25.5 percent of our sample compared to 22.9 percent of the nonsampled group.

Prevalences of Parasite-Tested Persons Missed by Economic Survey

In Cul-de-Sac, during the several-month interval between the parasitological and economic household surveys, changes of household occupancy caused roughly 11 percent of those tested on the parasitological survey to be omitted from the economic survey household rosters. With respect to health bias, various hypotheses are plausible: one might hypothesize, for example (1) that the persons missed were particularly healthy, having had sufficient initiative to move to better jobs outside the valley or even outside St. Lucia; or (2) that they were particularly sick, being so seriously disabled as to be hospitalized, or even to have died during the interval between the two surveys.[6] Another possibility, which we judge most likely of all, is that (3) these people are of average health conditions and have simply migrated to other houses in the valley. We do know from independent evidence that there is substantial shifting of people among houses, especially among unmarried adults.

In Table F.8, the parasite prevalence of those with matching economic survey data are compared to those for whom matching economic survey data were not obtained. We find that persons missed by the economic survey had a significantly higher (.01 level) prevalence of one parasite, *Trichuris*—68.1 percent vs. 57.0 percent—than persons included on the economic survey.[7] The prevalence differences for the other four parasites,

6. During 1960–1965 only 22 of 6,334 deaths in St. Lucia were registered as caused by schistosomiasis. Peter Jordan, noting that existing evidence does not indicate that schistosomiasis is being undercertified as a cause of death, concluded that schistosomiasis can hardly be considered a major cause of death at this stage [120] [143].

7. Since our concern is with the possibility that those listed may be *more* infected than those included in our sample, single-tail significance tests were used where those missed had a higher prevalence and two-tail tests where those missed had a lower prevalence.

Table F.8. Parasitological Prevalences Among Persons for Whom Economic Data Were and Were Not Obtained in Cul-de-Sac Valley (Ages 2 Years and Above), 1967–1968

Population	Persons tested	Persons found to have each parasite					
		Schisto- soma	Hook- worm	*Ascaris*	*Trichuris*	*Strongy- loides*	All parasite average[a]
Parasitological survey[b]	2,685	39.6%	55.4%	47.0%	58.2%	14.6%	43.0%
Economic survey[c]	2,397	40.2	55.3	47.3	57.0	14.7	42.9
Noneconomic survey[d]	288	35.1	56.6	44.8	68.1	13.5	43.8

[a] The average prevalence of all five parasites in the grouping.
[b] All persons for whom parasitological data were obtained.
[c] All persons for whom economic data were obtained in addition to parasitological data.
[d] All persons for whom economic data were not obtained but parasitological data were.

though, are not significant at the .10 level, however, either individually or for the five-parasite average.

Geest Worker Productivity Study

Our efforts to collect parasitological data from Geest workers for the Cul-de-Sac banana estate productivity study were conducted over a sixteen-month period—December 1967 to April 1969—during which time the personnel constituting the Geest labor force changed continually. Our list of candidates for testing consisted of those 810 workers for whom we had already obtained productivity data, specifically all those who had worked for Geest at any time during the period January 1966–June 1967. A large proportion of the persons worked for Geest only briefly. Others, apparently, drifted in and out of the Geest labor force, whose current size averaged quite close to 400 workers (Table F.9). It is estimated that approximately 500 of the workers on our productivity list remained in the Geest labor force during the period when we collected parasitological data from Geest workers. Thus, the 466 workers who provided stool speci-

Table F.9. Geest Worker Survey Sample Size, 1967–1969

Approximate Geest Cul-de-Sac Estate current labor force	400
Number of workers in productivity data sample (compiled from pay-cards of all who worked at any time between January 1966–June 1967)	810
Approximate number of workers from productivity data sample in Cul-de-Sac Estate labor force during parasitological testing period	500
Total productivity list workers with one or more stool returns	466

mens for analysis (Table F.9) represent about 90 percent of those workers on our candidate list[8] who were approached for testing.

Because of the prolonged period during which clinical examinations and stool-collection surveys were conducted,[9] temporary absence from work was effectively excluded as a cause of nonrespondence. The reasons for unwillingness of workers to attend the clinical exams (which were given during working hours without loss of pay to participating workers) and the reasons for unwillingness to provide stool specimens for analysis are undoubtedly varied; a frequently voiced reason, however, was the perceived intrusion into personal affairs. Impressionistically, the nonrespondents (less than 10 percent of the Geest work force) appeared to be a less "docile" group than the cooperants. The Geest overseer at Cul-de-Sac (a respected St. Lucian who had "risen from the ranks") admonished recalcitrants to cooperate. Noncooperation, consequently, involved an element of self-assertion. There is no evidence, however, as to whether the parasite-prevalence or intensity rates varied significantly between respondents and nonrespondents.

We are also concerned whether Geest workers have infection levels that are representative of (and, in particular, not lower than) other rural persons who are not in the Geest labor force. In Tables F.10–F.13 we compare the parasitic prevalences of Geest workers to other Cul-de-Sac Valley residents. It should be emphasized that we are *not* concerned with comparative prevalence levels, per se, but rather with intensity levels which *may*, to some extent, be proxied by group prevalence levels. The question, to repeat, is whether our sampled group was less severely affected by parasite infections than was the nonsampled population.

In order to learn more about the possibility that the persons excluded from the Geest labor force were victims of relatively high parasitic infection levels, we utilized our household survey data to compare Geest worker prevalences to prevalences of unemployed persons,[10] and also to prevalences among other (non-Geest) employed persons. Because it is likely that females are unemployed for numerous reasons unrelated to health, the comparisons are mostly in terms of the male population.[11]

8. Eighteen workers, not on our candidate list, provided stools without prior invitation, resulting in a tested-worker total of 484.

9. The clinical exams were conducted, intermittently, during December 1967 to September 1968. The stool-collection survey continued until mid-April 1969.

10. The unemployed are those who indicated no work activity on the economic survey, that is, they were neither employed by others nor working on their own.

11. To insure a homogeneous test universe, only the parasitological results obtained in the household survey are utilized (that is, none of the Geest on-site parasitological data are included).

Is the Geest work force a biased sample, with respect to parasite infection, of working-age adults? Table F.10 shows the percentages of persons in each of six population groups who were infected with each of the five parasites, and, in the last column, the average prevalence of the five parasites for all the people in each group. These overall prevalence statistics conceal, however, the differing age structures of the groups. This is important because overall prevalence rates are a function of the population age distribution, as we have already seen in Table F.3.[12]

Table F.11 shows, in columns 1 to 2, the relative age structures for three of the six groups in Table F.10 (groups 4–6), and, in columns 3–8,

Table F.10. Parasite Prevalences of Geest Workers Compared to Other Persons in Cul-de-Sac Valley (Ages 15–64), 1967–1968

Class	Persons tested	Persons found to have each parasite					
		Schisto-soma	*Hook-worm*	*Ascaris*	*Trichuris*	*Strongy-loides*	All parasite average[a]
(1) All economic survey	1,170	41.8%	68.5%	41.5%	50.3%	19.0%	44.2%
(2) All Geest	221	58.8	68.3	41.6	44.3	27.2	48.1
(3) Economic survey males	509	41.7	74.1	38.9	46.2	24.6	45.1
(4) Geest males	119	56.3	71.4	38.7	34.5	28.6	45.9
(5) Non-Geest employed males	319	30.7	77.7	36.7	47.3	30.0	43.9
(6) Males not employed	71	66.2	62.0	49.3	60.6	7.0	49.0

Note: The prevalence statistics in the table are from the household survey.
  [a] The average prevalence of all five parasites in the grouping.

provides a disaggregation, by age, of the parasite-prevalence rates for these groups. In the comparisons between Geest male workers and non-Geest employed males we find that, for *Schistosoma*, Geest males actually have a *higher* overall prevalence—56.3 percent vs. 30.7 percent (significant at the .01 level, see also Table F.12) and significantly higher prevalences (.10 level and .05 level) in three individual age groups. Geest males have a *lower* overall prevalence of *Trichuris*—34.5 percent vs. 47.3 percent (significant at the .05 level)—with the prevalence for the Geest males also significantly lower (.05 level) in two individual age groups. Though Geest males have a significantly *lower* prevalence in a single age group for hookworm and for *Ascaris*, the overall prevalence difference is not significant (.10 level) in either instance. The overall prevalence average

12. One might hypothesize that high prevalence of schistosomiasis is more seriously debilitating for older persons than for younger persons, because infected older persons may, on the average, have been infected for a longer period of time, with consequent greater likelihood of organ damage.

Table F.11. Age and Age-Prevalence Structures for Geest Worker Males, Non-Geest Employed Males, and Unemployed Males, 1967–1968

Age	Occupation class	Population		Persons found to have each parasite					
		Size	Percentage of class total	Schisto- soma	Hook- worm	Ascaris	Trichuris	Strongy- loides	All para- site average[a]
		(1)	(2)	(3)	(4)	(5)	(6)	(7)	(8)
15–19 years	Geest	18	15.1%	66.7%	72.2%	27.8%	44.4%	16.7%	45.6%
	Non-Geest	31	9.7	45.2	83.9	54.8	54.8	25.8	52.9
	Unemployed	49	69.0	69.4	59.2	51.0	65.3	10.2	51.0
20–24	Geest	4	3.4	50.0	75.0	75.0	0.0	25.0	45.0
	Non-Geest	28	8.8	42.9	92.9	28.6	35.7	25.0	45.0
	Unemployed	4	5.6	25.0	50.0	75.0	100.0	0.0	50.0
25–29	Geest	16	13.5	62.5	75.0	43.8	43.8	25.0	50.0
	Non-Geest	39	12.2	33.3	74.4	41.0	38.5	10.3	39.5
	Unemployed	1	1.4	100.0	0.0	0.0	100.0	0.0	40.0
30–34	Geest	16	13.5	62.5	87.5	43.8	37.5	31.3	52.5
	Non-Geest	36	11.3	22.2	66.7	47.2	52.8	27.8	43.3
	Unemployed	2	2.8	50.0	100.0	50.0	0.0	0.0	40.0
35–39	Geest	11	9.2	36.4	90.9	45.5	54.6	27.3	50.9
	Non-Geest	39	12.2	30.8	89.7	38.5	69.2	28.2	48.2
	Unemployed	2	2.8	50.0	50.0	0.0	0.0	0.0	20.0
40–44	Geest	16	13.5	67.5	50.0	43.8	18.8	37.5	42.5
	Non-Geest	43	13.5	27.9	69.8	46.5	53.5	20.9	43.7
	Unemployed	2	2.8	50.0	50.0	100.0	50.0	0.0	50.0
45–49	Geest	15	12.6	53.3	46.7	33.3	33.3	26.7	38.7
	Non-Geest	40	12.5	20.0	75.0	27.5	37.5	32.5	38.5
	Unemployed	0	0.0	—	—	—	—	—	—
50–64	Geest	23	19.3	47.8	78.3	30.4	26.1	34.8	43.5
	Non-Geest	63	19.8	30.2	76.2	20.6	49.2	38.1	42.9
	Unemployed	11	15.5	72.7	81.8	36.4	45.5	0.0	47.3
Total	Geest	119	100	56.3	71.4	38.7	34.5	28.6	45.9
	Non-Geest	319	100	30.7	77.7	36.7	47.3	30.0	43.9
	Unemployed	71	100	66.2	62.0	49.3	60.5	7.0	49.0

[a] The average prevalence of all five parasites in the age group.

of all parasites counted equally is slightly *higher* for Geest males than for other employed males—45.9 percent vs. 43.9 percent—but this difference is also not significant. Thus, Geest male workers do not appear to be unrepresentative, in terms of parasitic-infection levels, of other employed males.

Turning to the comparison of Geest male workers and unemployed males, we note, in column 2 of Table F.11, that there is considerable dissimilarity between the age distribution of these two groups. Unemployed males have very high relative representation in the 15–19 years age group —69.0 percent of the unemployed males vs. 15.1 percent and 9.7 percent of the Geest males and non-Geest employed males, respectively. Because of the parasitic age specificity, this relative age structure bias of the unemployed males toward the 15–19 years age group will result, *ceteris paribus*, in higher overall prevalences of *Schistosoma, Ascaris,* and *Trichuris* for the unemployed males.

Table F.12. Significance Test Results of Parasite-Prevalence Comparisons between Geest Male Workers and Non-Geest Employed Males, 1967–1968

Age	Schistosoma	Hookworm	Ascaris	Trichuris	Strongy-loides	All parasite average[a]
15–19 years			−*			
20–24						
25–29	+*					
30–34	+**					
35–39						
40–44				−**		
45–49	+**	−**				
50–64				−**		
Total	+***			−**		

Note: Since our concern is with the possibility that Geest workers are *less* infected than non-Geest employed workers, a single-tail test was applied in all instances where the Geest worker prevalence was the lower prevalence in the comparison and a two-tail test where the Geest prevalence was the higher prevalence. Thus, in comparing the numbers of minuses and pluses (indicating significantly lower and higher Geest prevalences, respectively) in the table, it should be recognized that the pluses (significantly higher Geest worker prevalences) were determined by a more conservative criterion than were the minuses.

[a] The average prevalence of all parasites in the age group.
−* = Geest worker prevalence lower than non-Geest worker prevalence at .10 significance level or better (single-tail test).
+* = Geest worker prevalence higher than non-Geest worker prevalence at .10 significance level or better (two-tail test).
** = .05 significance level.
*** = .01 significance level.

Should, then, the overall prevalence rates of the unemployed males be discounted for their age-structure bias? The answer depends upon a judgment as to whether the age structure of the unemployed males is exogenous or endogenous to our parasitic-infection/health-status/behavior system, that is, is the relative age structure a consequence of health conditions? If the age structure is exogenously determined—with, for example (as appears likely), teenagers finding entry into the labor force difficult due to immaturity or inexperience—we do want to discount the age-structure bias of the overall prevalences. On the other hand, if the age-structure bias is endogenous to the parasitic-infection/health-status/behavior system— with, for example, the high representation of unemployed males in the 15–19 years group being the *result* of parasite infection and consequent debilitation—we would consider the overall prevalences appropriate comparative statistics, without adjustment of the age distribution.

For help in resolving this issue, we must look at the relative parasite prevalences within the individual age groups. Thus, if high parasitic in-fection is a *cause* of unemployment, we will expect the unemployed to have significantly higher prevalences within individual age groups—espe-cially the 15–19 years age group, where the unemployed are concen-trated.

Table F.13, based on data in Table F.11, shows that there are few sig-nificant differences in age-specific prevalence rates between the Geest males and the unemployed males. The unemployed have a significantly higher prevalence of *Ascaris* overall—49.3 percent vs. 38.7 percent—and also in the 15–19 years age group—51.0 percent vs. 27.8 percent. The prevalence of *Trichuris* is also significantly higher for the unemployed males—60.5 percent vs. 34.5 percent—but the difference is not significant in any in-dividual age group.

Geest males, on the other hand, have a higher *Strongyloides* prevalence rate than the unemployed males for the 20–44 years group—30.2 percent vs. 0.0 percent (different at the .10 significance level) and for the 50–64

Table F.13. Significance Test Results of Parasite-Prevalence Comparisons between Geest Male Workers and Unemployed Males, 1967–1968

Age	*Schistosoma*	Hookworm	*Ascaris*	*Trichuris*	*Strongy-loides*	All parasite average[a]
15–19 years			— *			
20–44[b]					+ *	
50–64					+ *	
Total			— *	— ***	+ ***	

Note: Since our concern is with the possibility that Geest workers are *less* infected than unemployed persons, a single-tail test was applied in all instances where the Geest worker prevalence was the lower prevalence in the comparison and a two-tail test where the Geest prevalence was the higher prevalence. Thus, in comparing the numbers of minuses and pluses (indicating significantly lower and higher Geest prev-alences, respectively) in the table, it should be recognized that the pluses (signifi-cantly higher Geest worker prevalences) were determined by a more conservative criterion than were the minuses.

  [a] The average prevalence of all parasites in the age group.

  [b] Due to the very small unemployed population sizes in the individual age group-ings of the 20–44 years age range, a single aggregate grouping was utilized for signifi-cance testing. Since there were no unemployed persons in the 45–49 years age range, this grouping is excluded.

  — * = Geest worker prevalence lower than unemployed prevalence at .10 significance level or better (single-tail test).

  + * = Geest worker prevalence higher than unemployed prevalence at .10 signifi-cance level or better (two-tail test).

  *** = .01 significance level.

years group—34.8 percent vs. 0.0 percent (different at the .10 significance level)—as well as overall—28.6 percent vs. 7.0 percent (different at the .01 significance level). The higher overall average prevalence of the unemployed for all parasites combined (and weighted equally)—49.0 percent vs. 45.9 percent—is not significant. All in all, the evidence does not provide support for the hypothesis that our Geest worker sample is unrepresentative of adult males who are not in the labor force.

Dimensions, Ltd., Labor-Productivity Study

Our study at Dimensions, Ltd., deals with the all-female labor force of an urban firm. The workers were predominantly from the capital city, Castries, although some had "suburban" and rural addresses. Most of the girls were in the 16–25 years age range, in which, if the rural Cul-de-Sac age-prevalence pattern held (see Table F-3), the prevalence of schistosomiasis is particularly high. In terms of overall parasitic infection (on an equal weighting basis), this age group has an above-average infection rate.

We sought to include the total Dimensions, Ltd., labor force in our study. The response rate to the clinical examinations and the stool-collection effort was, in fact, quite high: only 3 of 162 girls employed did not attend the clinicals.[13] Stool-specimen containers were distributed to 100 percent of the work force, with second containers supplied to those who claimed loss, or who were otherwise dilatory. Stool specimens were returned by 150 girls (92.6 percent).[14] Reasons for nonresponse are probably similar to those experienced at Geest and are not considered likely to be health related.

The Schoolchildren Studies: Island-Wide and Babonneau Surveys

The two schoolchildren studies—the island-wide study and the Babonneau study—tested children in specific grades, children who were attending

13. Of these, one was absent from work, due to having a baby, and another was visiting her boyfriend at the hospital. The absence of the third person was not explained; however a stool specimen was obtained from this person.

14. The actual number of persons in the Dimensions, Ltd., productivity study is 114. This is less than the 150 who provided stool specimens, because (1) the limited capacity of laboratories in St. Lucia caused the analysis of some stools to be performed too late for inclusion in our study; and (2) the numbers of girls performing some jobs was so small that adequate sample sizes could not be obtained.

school during the respective testing periods. The studies obviously exclude both those who were not enrolled in school, and those who—although enrolled—were not tested due to absence.

Estimates based on the 1960 census for St. Lucia indicate that, in 1961, approximately 87 percent of primary schoolage children in St. Lucia were enrolled in school [176]. Actual attendance on the specific days that the island-wide survey was administered in the various schools was 81.7 percent of the estimated total enrollment for the grades surveyed. Although exact statistics regarding exclusions from the Babonneau study due to absenteeism are not available—these data had been obtained by the Research and Control Department prior to commencement of the economic study of the schoolchildren—these children were surveyed over a period of time, so that absenteeism on a single day would not have meant exclusion from the study. (Note that number of days absent is a variable used in the Babonneau study.) In the island-wide survey, as noted in chapter 5, stool specimens were returned by 158 of the 162 children (97.5 percent) who were selected, on a random sampling basis, from those in attendance on the survey day.

We lack detailed data on the causes of both nonenrollment and absenteeism, and therefore we cannot be certain that the health characteristics of the children included in our studies are representative of those excluded. It is our impression, however, that *non*attendance at school in St. Lucia is largely due to reasons other than ill-health. Children are, for example, frequently kept home from school to assist in the "heading" (carrying) of bananas to the buying points on banana-harvest days.[15] Moreover, the generally casual attitude of some St. Lucians toward school attendance has been noted by others: For example,

A seven year old boy living on an estate some twenty-five minutes downhill walking distance (for him) from Soufriere, attended school during the six months that I knew him about 60% of the time. Some days he had a "cold;" some days he had a sore toe; some days he had to help someone with this or that; and some days, insofar as I could determine, he stayed home because he had already been home so much that week that it did not seem worthwhile to go just for Friday—or even just for Thursday and Friday. On visits to rural areas I regularly encountered schoolchildren who were being kept home for reasons more or less inadequate by our standards—such as to help their mothers care for younger children, or for illnesses having neither signs nor symptoms. [169]

15. In one school, which was visited on a banana-harvest day during the island-wide survey, there was 100 percent absenteeism. The results of this obviously ill-timed visit are reflected in the 18.3 percent overall absenteeism figure encountered by the island-wide survey.

Conclusion

No simple summary can be made of all of the findings in this appendix. There appears to be scant evidence, however, to support the hypothesis that our samples are systematically biased in favor of uninfected and "healthy" persons.

Appendix G

WAGE-RATE CHANGES
AND THE SUPPLY OF LABOR

One of the most widely held views concerning the behavior of unskilled workers in less-developed countries is that they tend to work less when their wage-rates are increased.[1] More precisely, the hypothesis is that if the wage-rate is calculated on an hourly or daily basis, individuals work fewer hours per day or days per week when the wage-rate rises, whereas if a piece-rate system exists, workers complete fewer pieces of work per period when the piece-rate increases. A special form of this backward-bending labor-supply hypothesis is that workers reduce the quantity of labor supplied by the same proportion as the increases in rate of pay, continuing to earn a particular "target" income.

There is nothing "irrational" or indeed unusual about individual backward-bending labor-supply curves. Many individuals in developed countries who can freely determine their hours of work choose to work less when their rate of pay per unit of time rises. The pressures for longer vacations, more holidays, and a shorter work week that are almost universal among organized workers in developed and developing countries are another manifestation of this type of labor supply. But if less labor is offered in response to higher wages, this can act as a significant impediment to private and governmental efforts to achieve higher aggregate market output.

1. For a survey of the literature discussing this view, see [2].

Reliable data with which to test the backward-bending supply-curve hypothesis are notoriously scarce in less-developed nations, and the actual nature of supply-curve relationships in these countries is still a matter of considerable dispute. Fortunately, the work records of the Geest estate in Cul-de-Sac provide an excellent opportunity to test this general hypothesis as well as the specific target worker hypothesis. Task-work records were available both before and after an increase, in 1964, in the piece-rate for "carrying" bananas. Carrying is a task job that is generally performed only two days per week and only by women; it involves carrying stems of cut bananas from the trees to central collecting areas. Workers performing the carrying task now have the ability—within broad limits—to determine the number of stems they carry each hour, as well as the number of hours they work each day. As part of a general increase in wages negotiated with the union representing the workers, the wage rate per stem was increased in October 1964 from $.02 to $.03 (E.C.). Carrying was the only piece-rate job whose rate was increased at this time.

It is possible, however, that the increase in piece rate set by the Geest Company was above what was required, and that, as a result, an excess supply of labor was brought forth when the wage was increased. If this were the case, and if Geest hired some of the additional workers who were willing to work at the increased rate of pay, then a comparison of the mean number of stems carried per worker at the old and the new wage would be a downward-biased estimate of the true supply response. This conclusion would also hold if the comparison were restricted to those workers who were employed during both periods, for even their observed labor-supply behavior would be negatively affected by the entry of new workers.

Thus, the empirical analysis that follows provides an estimate of the average worker's labor-supply response to an increase in the wage rate under the assumption that the increased rate of pay was the increase required to bring forth the desired increase in aggregate labor supply.

The response to this piece-rate increase in terms of average number of stems carried per day and average daily earnings for two subestates in Cul-de-Sac is summarized in Table G.1.[2] Since the nature of the terrain and the average distance that the stems must be carried differ considerably between the two subestates, the results for the subestates should be viewed as separate tests of the hypothesis. The table indicates that the daily average of stems carried did not fall on La Pointe for the first carrying day each week but did decline significantly (at the .01 level) for the

---

2. It would also have been interesting to test the response of workers in terms of average number of hours worked per day, but such data were not available.

Table G.1. Output and Earnings Before and After Change in Piece Rate for Carrying Bananas, Two St. Lucian Estates, 1964

Estate and time interval	Mean (and standard deviation), number of stems carried per person			Mean (and standard deviation), earnings per person ($E.C.)		
	Carrying day of week					
	First	Second	Total	First	Second	Total
La Pointe Estate						
Before (12 weeks preceding rate change)	54	99	153	$1.13	$2.14	$3.27[a]
(N = 141)	(22)	(34)		(.53)	(.78)	
After (18 weeks following rate change)	57	78	135	$1.73	$2.42	$4.15
(N = 419)	(28)	(30)		(.88)	(.99)	
Crownlands Estate						
Before (11 weeks preceding rate change)	125	121	246	$2.86	$2.77	$5.63
(N = 118)	(64)	(55)		(1.48)	(1.24)	
After (32 weeks following rate change)	102	107	209	$3.22	$3.35	$6.57
(N = 350)	(54)	(40)		(1.70)	(1.35)	

[a] The average number of stems carried multiplied by the piece rate does not equal average earnings because bonuses are paid to compensate for especially long carrying distances. It is interesting to note that the amount by which earnings exceeded their base levels declined slightly after the wage increase—a fact indicating that the actual piece-rate increase was not quite 50 percent.

second carrying day, and declined significantly (at the .05 level) for the two days combined. On the Crownlands estate the average number of bunches carried declined significantly on each day (.01 level). Average daily earnings, however, rose for both days and on both estates.[3]

The data support the hypothesis that the labor-supply curves of St. Lucian estate-workers were backward-bending at the time; a 50 percent wage rise was accompanied by a 12 percent and 17 percent decline in the average number of stems carried per worker per week on La Pointe and Crownlands, respectively. However, the evidence does not support the "target worker" hypothesis, since the 50 percent wage increase was not offset by the decrease in number of stems carried; total weekly earnings per worker rose 27 percent on La Pointe and 17 percent on Crownlands.

3. Breaking the periods before and after the piece-rate increase into various subperiods did not alter the response-pattern reported in Table G.1. Extending the post-wage-increase period another three months, as was done in the Crownlands case, also did not change the general nature of piece-rate increase pattern.

Two possibilities, however, should be checked before the results can be regarded as an acceptable test of these hypotheses. First, the wage rise could, conceivably, have coincided with a temporary production cutback to which the estate managers responded by reducing the daily amount of work to be done by each worker rather than by reducing the number of workers employed in carrying bananas. In fact, this was not the case. Examination of data for the total number of bananas carried per week for each of the two carrying days (not shown in the tables) indicates that the total volume of work done actually increased after the wage increase for both days at both subestates.

The second point concerns the change in the composition of the work force after the wage increase. Since total output increased while the amount carried per worker decreased, it follows that additional workers were employed in the carrying activity. It is possible that these workers were less productive than those previously employed, and that output per worker for those previously engaged in carrying activities did not decline. In order to test for this possibility, a sample of those workers who were employed in the carrying operation both before and after the wage increase was selected and their productivity pattern investigated. As Table G.2 shows, the average number of bananas carried by workers in this group also decreased after the wage increase. Furthermore, there were no significant differences between the mean number of banana stems carried by persons in this group as compared with the total group considered in Table G.1, for either day on either estate, before and after the wage rate change.

Table G.2. Task Performance Before and After Change in Piece Rate for Carrying Bananas, for Those Workers Employed in Both Periods, Two St. Lucian Estates, 1964

| | Average number (and standard deviation) of stems carried per person | | | |
| | La Pointe (N = 31) | | Crownlands (N = 22) | |
	First day	Second day	First day	Second day
Before	55	100	135	135
	(23)	(35)	(70)	(56)
After	54	74	120	122
	(26)	(30)	(61)	(41)

Note: For La Pointe the decline in the mean number of stems carried before and after was—as in the case of the total sample—not significant for the first day but was significant for the second day. For Crownlands the decline was not significant for either day.

Appendix H

ECONOMIC CHANGE
AS A CAUSE OF DISEASE

While this book focuses on the effects of disease on economic development, this appendix deals with some possible effects of development on disease.[1] Increasing attention has recently been directed to the possibility that developmental activities—for example, the U.A.R.'s Aswan High Dam project[2]—may themselves expand disease. This appendix investigates the hypothesis that the expansion of banana cultivation on St. Lucia after 1950 was a causal factor in the spread of schistosomiasis on the island. This is one case of a more general class of cases in which the process of economic change contributes to environmental health problems.

The expansion of the St. Lucian banana industry and the accelerating displacement of sugar cane cultivation by bananas in the late 1950s has already been described in chapter 3. The decade of the 1950s was also noted, in chapter 4, to have witnessed the apparent spread of schistosomiasis in St. Lucia. The seemingly explosive rise in prevalence of that

1. A much more detailed treatment of the material in this appendix may be found in [38, ch. 11].

2. As noted in chapter 1, it is feared that the Aswan High Dam, by greatly extending the perennial irrigation of arid regions, may allow a large expansion in the potential habitats of the intermediate snail host for schistosomiasis. In 1937, following the introduction three years previously of perennial irrigation into four areas of Egypt in connection with the original, low dam at Aswan, geometric increases in schistosomiasis were observed [147]. See also [115] [116] [122] [133] [154].

disease during the 1950s,[3] after confinement to small foci since its discovery on St. Lucia in 1924, has suggested the "trigger-hypothesis"—the idea that some critical socio-economic parameter must have shifted to unleash the infection.[4]

Though we hypothesize that expansion of the banana industry was a causal factor in the spread of schistosomiasis, the specific nature of the suspected causal linkage is not obvious. While drainage ditches flanking the rows of banana plants on the large valley-floor estates constitute one of several habitat types for the intermediate snail host in the schistosome life-cycle/transmission process, schistosomiasis researchers question whether the banana drains have been a major force in overall transmission [101]. The actual linkage might be circuitous, related, perhaps, to various changes in sociological patterns—possibly effected by the exchange of a seasonal crop (sugar cane), which entailed migratory labor movements, for a nonseasonal crop (bananas).

Data to test directly the causal linkage hypothesis are not available. Thus, the hypothesis is only inferentially tested—using cross-sectional rather than time-series data for the period of expanded banana cultivation and disease prevalence; the data used involve current schistosomal-infection rates for persons who are, and are not, working at banana cultivation. If persons involved in banana cultivation have greater prevalence of schistosomiasis, *ceteris paribus,* then we will regard this as supporting the hypothesis that expansion of banana production led to increased disease prevalence.

The Data

Data are from our economic survey and the associated parasitological survey for the 1,060 households in the Cul-de-Sac Valley of St. Lucia. From the occupational responses to the economic survey, two groups associated with banana cultivation are identified: (1) employees of the large (nine hundred acres) Geest banana plantation, and (2) private

3. There might be a bias in the data for the period, which are based on routine stool examinations. It is possible that the infection became widespread earlier, but was only gradually recognized during the 1950s. Alternative evidence, however, supports the view that the infection only recently became widespread [97].

4. Suggested "trigger" hypotheses relating to the sudden spread of the schistosomal infection from the early transmission foci include: the occurrence of fires which largely destroyed Castries (1948) and Soufriere (1954), resulting in large-scale population movements; the physical facilitation of population movement with the construction of the road linking Castries and Soufriere (1955) ; and educational expansion which, by bringing large groups of children together, might have offered increased opportunities for transmission.

banana growers working generally small holdings (usually less than five acres and often less than a single acre).

The private-banana-grower group is distinguished from the Geest plantation workers by the fact that it is not known which members of private-grower households actually work the banana holding. Since it appears likely that many or all members of a household may work on the holding or, at least, experience extensive physical contact with it, all members of the private-grower households are included in the private-grower group. The private-grower holdings in Cul-de-Sac Valley also are topographically differentiated from the valley-floor Geest estate. Located on hillsides, the relatively small private holdings generally lack the formal drainage ditch systems (habitat of the intermediate snail host of the schistosomal infection) of the Geest estate. Thus the private-grower holdings would appear to be an inferior source for schistosomiasis transmission as compared with the Geest estate drainage system.

Hypothetical Model

It is hypothesized that persons associated with banana cultivation have a greater probability of becoming infected with schistosomiasis than persons not associated with banana cultivation. A priori sentiments, based on the above-described differentiation, suggest a stronger banana cultivation-schistosomiasis relationship—that is, a higher schistosomiasis-prevalence rate—for Geest estate workers than for private growers in Cul-de-Sac Valley.

From the hypothesis that banana cultivation, particularly on the valley-floor estate, contributes to schistosomiasis transmission, there follows a corollary hypothesis that those having direct access to these primary transmission foci will cause development of secondary transmission foci for the spread of the schistosomal infection to the rest of the population. Thus, we expect to find that banana estate workers, having developed a high schistosomiasis prevalence level due to their access to primary transmission sites, will subsequently export the infection to their household neighborhoods, where secondary transmission sites will develop. Presuming patterns of social interaction to bear an inverse distance rule, we hypothesize that schistosomiasis prevalence among persons not engaged in banana cultivation will diminish with their distance from estate worker households.

The analyses of our hypotheses are principally conducted through statistical significance tests of differences in schistosomiasis prevalence for groups that are differentiated by whether or not they are engaged in banana cultivation and by distance from banana estate worker households. Caution is advisable, however, because we cannot be certain that prevalence differences between these groups reflect only the effects of banana cultivation. Moreover, there is a complex causation issue here regarding whether the observed prevalence variations within nonbanana cultivation groups—according to age, sex, and household area—are really independent of the hypothesized banana-cultivation influence on schistosomal infection. This potential nonindependence appears most serious for the household-area factor: thus, if high-prevalence banana cultivators live in household neighborhoods where the nonbanana cultivators also have high prevalences (a circumstance generally found for the Cul-de-Sac data), transmission causality may run in either, or both, directions. Consequently, some portion of the prevalence adjustments—for the age, sex, and household-area factors—performed in the following analyses may be inappropriate.

Geest Worker Prevalence Comparisons

Within the 15–79 year age range covering all workers on the Geest estate, 231 parasite-tested persons were identified by the economic survey as Geest workers [5] and 1,157 were indicated to be employed elsewhere or to be unemployed. The non-Geest workers, based on the stool-specimen results of the parasitological survey, had a schistosomiasis prevalence of 35.4 percent. The unadjusted Geest worker prevalence was 57.6 percent and the *adjusted* prevalence statistics for this group were between 53 percent and 59 percent, depending on the particular adjustment that was used. Even the 53 percent prevalence, however, is significantly greater (.01 level) [6] than the 35.4 percent schistosomiasis prevalence of the non-Geest workers.

---

5. Of the 231 persons identified as Geest workers in connection with the household survey, only 157 were positively matched to payroll records at Geest (for the purpose of the rural-productivity study described in chapter 5). Though the possibility of survey error exists, the lack of success in matching the residual 74 persons is more likely the result of the previously described proclivity of St. Lucians for name changing (chapter 3). Nevertheless the 157-member matched-worker subgroup had a somewhat higher schistosomiasis prevalence—60.5 percent—than the unmatched-worker subgroup—51.4 percent. (The difference in the age/sex/area-adjusted prevalence statistics for the two subgroups is only 1.3 percent—in favor of the matched workers.)

6. "Upper-tail" significance tests were used in all analyses in this appendix.

Private-Grower Prevalences

For comparability with the Geest worker group, the private-banana-grower household members were initially separated into an adult group (15–79 years) and a children's group (2–14 years).[7]

Generally the schistosomiasis prevalences of the private-grower groups were substantially below comparable Geest worker prevalences. The age/sex-adjusted prevalence statistic of adult private growers is 43.1 percent, compared to a 59.3 percent comparably adjusted prevalence for Geest workers. At the same time, the 43.1 percent adjusted prevalence statistic of the 275 adult private growers is significantly greater (.01 level) than the 32.8 percent prevalence among the 882 nonbanana cultivators (neither Geest nor private). The household-area adjustment, however, is negative and large, with the result that its inclusion reduces the age/sex/area-adjusted prevalence statistic for adult private growers to 34.3 percent; this is not significantly greater (even at the .10 level) than the 32.8 percent prevalence for persons not engaged in banana cultivation. A similar pattern of significantly different (at the .01 level) age/sex-adjusted prevalence statistics, but nonsignificance age/sex/*area*-adjusted prevalence statistics, was found for both the 346 children in the private-grower group and for the aggregated (2–79 years) group.

The Socio-Economic Status Factor

Socio-economic status—a factor which, *inter alia*, indicates housing conditions, level of sanitary facilities, hygienic standards, nutritional levels, etc.—is plausibly correlated with likelihood of infection [83]. Socio-economic stratification among Cul-de-Sac Valley households appears constrained to a relatively narrow band—insufficient, it would seem, to be a determinant of parasite-prevalence differences. Nevertheless, the hypothesis should be considered that the relatively high schistosomiasis prevalence of Geest workers is a consequence of relatively low socio-economic status, rather than an independent association with banana cultivation.

This hypothesis was investigated according to two approaches: (1) a

7. The 80+ years age group—representing ages above the Geest worker group and having a 33.3 percent schistosomiasis prevalence for only 21 persons in the group—was deleted for computational convenience. The under 2 years age group—with only 3.3 percent of the 180 persons in the group positive for schistosomiasis—was also deleted for statistical convenience, in consideration of the low infection rate of the group.

comparison of schistosomiasis prevalences by occupations, and (2) a Geest-non-Geest comparison of prevalences of other parasites.

In the first approach, estimates were made of the relative incomes for the various occupations indicated on the economic survey for the head of each Cul-de-Sac household (Geest and private-grower households excluded). Based on these estimates, the households were grouped and ranked in three occupational classes—"low," "intermediate," and "elite" —to test the hypothesis that the probability of schistosomal infection is a function of socio-economic stratification of the degree found in Cul-de-Sac. (The usual prevalence statistics were computed to standardize for dissimilar age, sex, and household-area distributions.)

Prevalence rates were compared for the 462-member "low" grouping and both the 46-member "elite" grouping and the aggregated 93-member "elite" plus "low" groupings (15–79 years age range only). The hypothesis that the higher socio-economic groupings would have lower schistosomiasis prevalences, however, was not supported by statistical tests for either comparison.

The second approach for testing whether socio-economic rank might be a factor in the relatively high schistosomiasis prevalences of Geest workers focused upon the comparative prevalences of other (nonschistosomiasis) parasites. It was assumed that if a socio-economic dichotomy between the Geest and non-Geest populations is the factor responsible for the large schistosomiasis-prevalence difference, it will similarly cause higher prevalences of other parasitic infections among Geest workers.

Of the four nonschistosomiasis helminths tested for on the parasitological survey, hookworm and *Strongyloides* are soil-transmitted and *Ascaris* and *Trichuris* are fecal-orally transmitted. Since the soil-transmission feature of hookworm and *Strongyloides* might involve an agricultural bias, only *Ascaris* and *Trichuris* were utilized for the Geest and non-Geest prevalence comparisons.

For the *Ascaris* infection, the age/sex-adjusted prevalence among Geest workers—44.8 percent—is significantly higher (.10 level) than the prevalence among non-Geest workers—39.9 percent. When the Geest worker prevalence is also adjusted for geographic area differences, however, the prevalence falls to 43.0 percent, and this is not significantly greater than the non-Geest prevalence rate. For the *Trichuris* infection, both the age/sex-adjusted and age/sex/area-adjusted prevalence statistics of the Geest group are lower (by about 8.5 percent) than the non-Geest-worker prevalence—52.9 percent—not higher, as hypothesized.

In summary, neither of the two test approaches has provided support for the hypothesis that a socio-economic factor contributed to the relatively high schistosomiasis prevalences of Geest workers.

Geest Worker Secondary Transmission Profile

As described above, a corollary hypothesis to our finding that Geest banana estate workers have higher schistosomiasis prevalences is that these workers will export the infection from the banana estates to the workers' household neighborhoods, where secondary foci establishment extend the infection to nonbanana cultivators. Consequently, we next test the hypothesis that an additional factor of schistosomiasis-prevalence determination is proximity to a Geest banana worker household.

A test of the proximity hypothesis was performed by classifying the Cul-de-Sac Valley non-Geest population according to household distance from the nearest Geest worker household. The proximity classification, derived from a field survey map of Cul-de-Sac showing the locations of the numbered households, includes five categories: (1) the Geest workers themselves; (2) the other members of Geest worker households; (3) the households of the "immediate neighborhood" (area 1); (4) the households of the "nonimmediate neighborhood" (area 2); and (5) the residual "nonneighborhood" households (area 3).[8] In computing the age, sex, and area adjustments to isolate the Geest proximity factor, the area 3 grouping was utilized as the standard in the adjustment formula.[9]

It was found from the data on schistosomiasis prevalence for these groups that prevalences generally declined with household distance from the Geest workers. Table H.1 shows the schistosomiasis prevalences for the nonprivate grower population of Cul-de-Sac, 2–79 years, classified according to distance from the nearest Geest banana worker household. Beginning with the Geest workers themselves and extending through the other members of their households and the households of areas 1, 2, and 3, the hypothesized pattern of prevalence decline with increasing distance is observed. Furthermore, most of the prevalence differences between proximity classss are statistically significant at levels varying between .10 and .01, depending on whether the age/sex-adjusted or age/sex/area-

8. Treating the Geest worker households as the foci of the secondary transmission model assumes that the true transmission foci (fresh water snail habitats) are near enough to the Geest worker households to yield, on the average, a sufficient approximation.

While scale measurements were utilized in classifying households according to Geest household proximity (area 1 perimeter = 150 yards, area 2 perimeter = 400 yards), the level of approximation of the household map requires that distance interpretations of the proximity groupings be limited to ordinality.

9. The area 3 proximity class is unlikely to be a totally unbiased background standard against which the secondary transmission effects of the Geest workers can be measured. Representing, however, the most distant households from the Geest households, the area 3 class is expected simply to be *least* biased.

Table H.1. Schistosomiasis Prevalences for Nonprivate Grower Population (2–79 Years), According to Household Distance from Geest Workers

Group	Total persons	Actual prevalence	Age/sex-adjusted prevalence	Age/sex/area-adjusted prevalence
Geest workers	231	57.6%	59.3%	56.7%*
Geest worker families	394	55.6	55.4***	50.9***
Area 1	310	45.2	45.2***	36.4***
Area 2	283	29.7	29.8**	26.0
Area 3	825	22.8	22.8ᵃ	22.8ᵃ

Note: Significance tests were performed only for the adjusted prevalence statistics.

  * Significantly higher prevalence (.10 level) than the next lower group (upper-tail test).

  ** Significantly higher prevalence (.05 level) than the next lower group (upper-tail test).

  *** Significantly higher prevalence (.01 level) than the next lower group (upper-tail test).

  ᵃ Area 3 actual prevalence.

adjusted statistics are utilized in the comparisons. It appears likely that causation predominantly runs from Geest worker infection to infection of the surrounding neighborhoods, rather than vice versa.

Private-Grower Prevalences Reviewed

The recognition of Geest worker household proximity as a factor influencing prevalence invites a reconsideration of the private-banana-grower analysis. Thus, the private-grower prevalence is now adjusted for a "proximity prevalence bias"—computed, according to the usual technique, by comparing the Geest-worker-household-proximity classification distributions of the private-grower and nonprivate grower/Geest worker groups. The application of this factor to the previously computed schisto-somiasis-prevalence statistics results in positive adjustments of 1.6 percent, 3.2 percent, and 2.5 percent for the adult, children's, and aggregated age groupings, respectively. For the new age/sex/proximity-adjusted prevalence statistic, the private-grower prevalence is significantly higher than the nonbanana cultivator (neither private nor Geest) prevalence (at the .01 level) for all three age groupings. With the inclusion of the household-area prevalence adjustment, the private-grower prevalence is not significantly higher for the adult grouping, but remains significantly higher (at the .05 level) for both the pre-adult and aggregated age groupings.

Summary

Workers on the Geest banana estate at Cul-de-Sac have been found to have significantly higher schistosomiasis prevalences than other workers, even after adjusting for other factors affecting prevalence—age, sex, and household region. Additional tests fail to support the hypothesis that a socio-economic factor might be the ultimate cause of the prevalence differences. A further series of prevalence comparisons for population groups classified according to household distance from the households of the Geest banana workers, showed that the Geest workers comprise the peaks of geographic prevalence "hills." The pattern of prevalence decline according to distance of nonbanana cultivators' households from the households of Geest workers is consistent with an epidemiological model in which high schistosomiasis prevalences for banana workers are acquired at foci on the banana estate, with subsequent transmission of the infection to nearby neighborhoods.

The epidemiological contribution of small, private banana growers, who lack the extensive drainage system-snail habitats of the estate, is less evident. The secondary transmission potential of these private growers appears overshadowed by that of the higher-prevalence Geest workers. It is possible that the estates are the only primary transmission foci: the slightly higher than average prevalences for private growers might be the result of many private growers having initially worked on the estates, prior to securing the necessary capital for cultivating bananas on their own account. In any event, the cross-sectional tests employed are, at best, only inferential tests of causation for the dynamic banana-cultivation extension and schistosomal-infection expansion processes which occurred during the 1950s on St. Lucia.

We have found evidence that expansion of banana cultivation in St. Lucia led to an increase in prevalence of schistosomiasis. If this causation has actually occurred, the policy implications depend upon the social and economic effects of schistosomiasis. Though current effects appear to be slight, future intensity levels, assuming transmission of the infection is allowed to continue unchecked, may bring appreciable losses. The findings reported here serve as a reminder that as economic-developmental planning is carried forward anywhere in the world, there is need to consider the possible consequences of the proposed developmental activities for the transmission of disease, and the subsequent secondary effects of disease on the economy.

REFERENCES

General Economics and Statistics

[1] American Child Health Association. Research Division. *A Health Survey of Eighty-Six Cities*. 2 vols. New York: The Association, 1923.

[2] Berg, E. J. "Backward-Sloping Labor Supply Functions in Dual Economies—The Africa Case." *Quarterly Journal of Economics* 75 (August 1961): 468–492.

[3] Bigelow, George H., and Herbert F. Lombard. *Cancer and Other Chronic Diseases in Massachusetts*. Boston: Houghton Mifflin Co., 1933.

[4] Blake, John B. "The Early History of Vital Statistics in Massachusetts." *Bulletin of the History of Medicine* 29 (January–February 1955): 46–68.

[5] Chadwick, Edwin. *Report on the Sanitary Conditions of the Labouring Population of Great Britain*. Edited with an introduction by M. W. Flinn. Edinburgh: University Press, 1965.

[6] Council of Hygiene Citizens Association. *Report on the Sanitary Condition of New York*. New York: D. Appleton Co., 1865.

[7] Denison, Edward Fulton. *The Sources of Economic Growth in the United States and the Alternatives Before Us*. Supplementary Paper no. 13. New York: Committee for Economic Development, 1962.

[8] Dublin, Louis I., and Jessamine Whitney. "On the Cost of Tuberculosis." *Journal of the American Statistical Association* 17 (1920–1921): 441–450.

[9] FAO. Committee on Commodity Problems. *Trade Patterns and Blocks in the World Banana Trade*. Rome: FAO, 1966.

[10] Farr, William. *Vital Statistics*. Edited by Noel A. Humphreys. London: The Sanitary Institute, 1885.

[11] Finney, D. J. *Probit Analysis*. Cambridge: Cambridge University Press, 1962.

[12] Goldberger, Arthur S. *Econometric Theory*. New York: John Wiley, 1964.

[13] Jorgenson, D. W., and Z. Griliches. "The Explanation of Productivity Change." *Review of Economic Studies* 34 (July 1967): 249–283.

[14] Marshall, Alfred. *Principles of Economics*. 8th ed. London: Macmillan, 1936. Bk. 4, ch. 5, p. 193.

[15] Marx, Karl. *Das Kapital*. Translated from 3d German ed. by Samuel Moore and Edward Aveling. Edited by Frederick Engels. New York: Random House, 1906. Ch. 10.

[16] Meier, Gerald M., and Robert E. Baldwin. *Economic Development*. New York: John Wiley, 1957. Pp. 319–324.

[17] Mill, John Stuart. *Principles of Political Economy*. London: J. W. Parker, 1848. P. 50.

[18] Petty, William. *Political Arithmetic*. London: R. Clavel, 1691.

[19] Rosen, George. "Problems in the Application of Statistical Analysis to the Questions of Health: 1700–1880." *Bulletin of the History of Medicine* 29 (January–February 1955): 27–45.

[20] Shattuck, Lemuel. *The Vital Statistics of Boston*. Philadelphia: Lea & Blanchard, 1841.

[21] Stolnitz, George J. "A Century of International Mortality Trends." *Population Studies* 9, pt. 1 (July 1955): 24–55, and 10, pt. 2 (July 1956): 17–42.

[22] Tobin, James. "The Application of Multivariate Probit Analysis to Economic Survey Data." Cowles Foundation discussion paper no. 1, Yale University, New Haven, Conn., December 1955. Mimeographed.

Health Economics

[23] Andersen, Stig. "Operations Research in Public Health." *Indian Journal of Public Health* 7 (October 1963): 141–151.

[24] Auster, Richard, Irving Leveson, and Deborah Saracheck. "The Production of Health, an Exploratory Study." *The Journal of Human Resources* 4 (Fall, 1969): 411–436.

[25] Barlow, Robin. "The Economic Effects of Malaria Eradication." *American Economic Review Papers and Proceedings* 57 (May 1967): 130–157.

[26] Barlow, Robin. *The Effects of Malaria Eradication*. Bureau of Public Health Economics, Research Series, no. 15. Ann Arbor, Mich.:

School of Public Health, University of Michigan, 1968.

[27] Coleman, Hubert A. "The Relationship of Socio-Economic Status to the Performance of Junior High School Students." *Journal of Experimental Education* 9 (September 1940): 61–63.

[28] Dublin, Louis I., and Alfred J. Lotka. *The Money Value of a Man.* New York: Ronald Press Co., 1946.

[29] Dunn, C. L. "The Economic Value of the Prevention of Disease." *Indian Journal of Economics* 4 (January 1924): 127–141.

[30] Enke, Stephen. "Public Health and Effective Labor." In *Economics for Development.* Englewood Cliffs, N.J.: Prentice-Hall, 1963. Pp. 398–414.

[31] Fein, Rashi. *Economics of Mental Illness: A Report to the Staff Director, Jack R. Ewalt.* Joint Commission on Mental Illness and Health Monograph, Series no. 2. New York: Basic Books, 1958.

[32] Fein, Rashi. "Health Programs and Economic Development." In *Economics of Health and Medical Care, Proceedings of the Conference May 10–12, 1962.* Ann Arbor, Mich.: University of Michigan, 1964. Pp. 271–281.

[33] Fisher, Irving. *Bulletin of the Committee of One Hundred on National Health, Being a Report on the National Vitality, Its Wastes and Conservation.* Prepared for the National Conservation Commission. Washington, D.C.: Government Printing Office, 1909.

[34] Fisher, Irving. "Economic Aspect of Lengthening Life." *American Health* 2 (March 1909): 8–9.

[35] Fuchs, Victor R. "Some Economic Aspects of Mortality in the United States." Unpublished manuscript, National Bureau of Economic Research, New York City, July 1965. Mimeographed.

[36] Hansen, W. Lee. "A Note on the Cost of Children's Mortality." *Journal of Political Economy* 55 (June 1957): 257–262.

[37] "Health and Economic Development, A Symposium." *Comparative Studies in Society and History, An International Quarterly* 8 (July 1966):
"On Health and Economic Development." Mark Perlman. Pp. 433–449.
"Comment on M. Perlman's Paper." R. Barlow. Pp. 449–451.
"Cholera in Nineteenth-Century Europe: A Tool for Social and Economic Analysis." C. E. Rosenberg. Pp. 452–463.
"Effects of Pestilence and Plague, 1315–85." J. C. Russell. Pp. 464–473.
"Plague Effects in Medieval Europe." S. L. Thrupp. Pp. 474–483.

[38] Helminiak, Thomas W. "The Sugar-Bananas Shift on St. Lucia, West Indies: Bilharzia and Malaria Disease Causal Linkages." Ph.D. dissertation, University of Wisconsin, 1971.

[39] Henderson, A. "The Cost of Children." *United Nations Department of Economics and Social Affairs Population Studies* 3 (September

1959) : 130–150.

[40]   Kaprio, Leo A. "The Economics of Health in Relationship to International Health Activities." Paper read before the Health Congress of the Royal Society of Health at Eastbourne, April 1965. Pp. 26–30. Typewritten. Available from author, W.H.O. Regional Office for Europe, Copenhagen.

[41]   Klarman, Herbert E. *The Economics of Health.* New York: Columbia University Press, 1965.

[42]   Klarman, Herbert E. "Measuring the Benefits of a Health Program —The Control of Syphilis." In *Measuring Benefits of Government Investments.* Edited by Robert Dorfman. Washington, D.C.: The Brookings Institution, 1963.

[43]   Knowles, James Christopher. "The Economic Effects of Health and Disease in an Underdeveloped Country." Ph.D. dissertation, University of Wisconsin, 1970.

[44]   Lawrence, P. S. "Chronic Illness and Socio-Economic Status." *Public Health Reports* 63 (1948) : 1507–1521.

[45]   Lee, F. S. *The Human Machine and Industrial Efficiency.* New York: Longmans, Green & Co., 1918.

[46]   Malenbaum, Wilfred. "Health and Productivity in Poor Areas." In *Empirical Studies in Health Economics: Proceedings.* Edited by Herbert E. Klarman. Baltimore: Johns Hopkins University Press, 1970.

[47]   Massachusetts Sanitary Commission (Lemuel Shattuck, et al.). *Report of a General Plan for the Promotion of Public and Personal Health.* Boston: Dutton and Wentworth, 1850.

[48]   Mountin, Joseph W. *Organized Health Services in a County of the United States.* Foreword by Milton I. Roemer and Ethel A. Wilson. Public Health Service Publication 197. Washington, D.C.: Federal Security Agency, 1951.

[49]   Mushkin, Selma J. "Health as an Investment." *Journal of Political Economy* 70 pt. 2, suppl. (October 1962) : 129–157.

[50]   Mushkin, Selma J., and Francis d'A. Collings. "Economic Costs of Disease and Injury." *Public Health Reports* 74 (1959) : 795–809.

[51]   Myrdal, G. "Economic Aspects of Health." *W.H.O. Chronicle* 6 (1952) : 203–218.

[52]   Newman, Peter. *Malaria Eradication & Population Growth: With Special Reference to Ceylon and British Guiana.* Graduate School of Public Health, University of Michigan. Ann Arbor, Mich.: Braun-Brumfield, 1965.

[53]   Ogburn, W. F. "The Financial Cost of Rearing a Child." In *Standards of Child Welfare,* edited by William L. Chenery. Sec. 1, Children's Bureau Conference Series No. 1. Washington, D.C.: U.S. Government Printing Office, 1919. Pp. 26–30.

[54] Pan American Health Organization, Advisory Committee on Medical Research. "Research Needs on the Economics of Health and Medical Care in Latin America." Document No. RES. 1/3, May 17, 1963. Pan American Union, Washington, D.C.

[55] Pan American Health Organization, Advisory Committee on Medical Research. "Research on the Economics of Health and Medical Care in Latin America." Document No. RES. 2/13, April 23, 1963. Pan American Union, Washington, D.C.

[56] Perlman, Mark. "Some Economic Aspects of Public Health Programs in Underdeveloped Areas." In *Economics of Health and Medical Care, Proceedings of the Conference, May 10–12, 1962.* Ann Arbor, Mich.: University of Michigan, 1964. Pp. 286–299.

[57] Perrott, G., and S. D. Collins. "Relation of Sickness to Income and Change in 10 Surveyed Communities." *Public Health Reports* 50 (1935): 595–622.

[58] Pettenkofer, Max Joseph. *The Value of Health to a City.* Two lectures delivered in 1873. Translated from the German with an introduction by Henry E. Sigerist. Baltimore: Johns Hopkins Press, 1941.

[59] Schlenker, Robert Erwin. "Health Improvements and Economic Growth: Neoclassical Theory and Puerto Rican Experience." Ph.D. dissertation, University of Michigan, 1968.

[60] U.S. Department of Health, Education, and Welfare. *Economic Benefits from Public Health Services.* PHS Publication no. 1178. Washington, D.C.: U.S. Government Printing Office, 1964.

[61] Weisbrod, Burton A. *Economics of Public Health: Measuring the Economic Impact of Diseases.* Philadelphia: University of Pennsylvania Press, 1961.

[62] Weisbrod, Burton A., and Selma Mushkin. "Investment in Health Expenditure—Lifetime Health Expenditures on the 1960 Work Force." In *Economics of Health and Medical Care, Proceedings of the Conference, May 10–12, 1962.* Ann Arbor, Mich.: University of Michigan, 1964. Pp. 257–270.

[63] W.H.O. "Assessment of the Economic Impact of Parasitic Diseases with Special Reference to Onchocerciasis: Report of an Informal Meeting of W. H. O. Advisers." W.H.O., Geneva, 1968, ONCHO/WP/68.8, p. 4. Mimeographed.

[64] W.H.O. *Measurement of Levels of Health.* W.H.O. Technical Report, series no. 137. Geneva: W.H.O., 1957.

[65] Winslow, C. E. A. *The Cost of Sickness and the Price of Health.* W.H.O. Monograph Series no. 7. Geneva: W.H.O., 1951.

[66] Wiseman, Jack. "Cost-Benefit Analysis and the Health Service Policy." *Scottish Journal of Political Economy* 10 (1963): 128–145.

[67] Woods, E. A., and C. B. Metzger. *America's Human Wealth: The Money Value of Human Life.* New York: F. S. Crofts, 1927.

Schistosomiasis and Other Diseases [1]

GENERAL

[68] *Dorland's Illustrated Medical Dictionary.* 23rd ed. Philadelphia: W. B. Saunders Co., 1957. P. 393.

[69] Farooq, M. "Recent Developments and Trends in Epidemiology and Control of Schistosomiasis." *The Journal of Tropical Medicine and Hygiene* 72 (1969): 210–211.

[70] Gelfand, M. "The Clinical Background." In *A Clinical Study of Intestinal Bilharziasis in Africa.* Edited by M. Gelfand. London: Edward Arnold Ltd., 1967. Pp. 1–15.

[71] Greenbaum, Leonard, ed. "Bilharziasis/Schistosomiasis." *Phoenix* 1 (December 1961): 1–5.

[72] Hunter, George W., W. Frye, and J. Clyde Swartzwelder. *A Manual of Tropical Medicine.* 4th ed. Philadelphia and London: W. B. Saunders Co., 1966.

[73] Jones, Arthur W. *Introduction to Parasitology.* Reading, Mass.: Addison-Wesley, 1967. P. 253.

[74] Jordan, Peter, and Gerald Webbe. *Human Schistosomiasis.* London: William Heinemann Medical Books, 1969.

[75] *W.H.O. Expert Committee on Bilharziasis, 3rd Report.* W.H.O. Technical Report Series, no. 299. Geneva: W.H.O., 1965.

[76] W.H.O. "Nature and Extent of the Problem of Bilharziasis." *W.H.O. Chronicle* 13 (January 1959): 3–19.

[77] Weir, John M. "The Unconquered Plague." *Bulletin of the Atomic Sciences* October 1966, pp. 46–48.

LIFE CYCLE AND EPIDEMIOLOGY

[78] Gelfand, M. "The Life Cycle in Man." In *A Clinical Study of Intestinal Bilharziasis in Africa.* Edited by M. Gelfand. London: Edward Arnold Ltd., 1967.

[79] Hairston, Nelson G. "Population Ecology and Epidemiological Problems." In *Ciba Foundation Symposium: Bilharziasis.* Edited by G. E. W. Wolstenholme and Maeve O'Connor. Boston: Little, Brown and Company, 1962. Pp. 36–62.

1. This section of the bibliography includes—in addition to those materials cited in the text—a small, purposeful sampling from the vast literature available on schistosomiasis. The selected items are offered to the interested reader who is not expert in his knowledge of schistosomiasis and who desires a greater familiarity with the subject in general and, especially, wth those aspects of the disease which relate to the problems faced in our study. Readers wishing to pursue the subject still more intensively are referred to the comprehensive *Schistosomiasis: A Bibliography of the World's Literature from 1852 to 1962,* by Kenneth S. Warren and Vaun A. Newill (Western Reserve University Press, 1967), and, for literature since 1962, to the National Library of Medicine's *Index Medicus* schistosomiasis listings.

[80] Hubendick, Bengt. "Factors Conditioning the Habitat of Fresh Water Snails." *Bulletin of W.H.O.* 18 (1958): 1072–1080.

[81] Oliver, L., and N. Ansari. "The Epidemiology of Bilharziasis." In *Bilharziasis: International Academy of Pathology.* Edited by F. K. Mostofi. New York: Springer-Verlag, 1967. Pp. 8–15.

[82] Sturrock, Robert F. "Pre-Control Studies in St. Lucia of *Biomphalaria glabrata* and *Schistosoma mansoni.*" Unpublished paper delivered at the Thirteenth Scientific Meeting of the Standing Advisory Committee for Medical Research in the British Caribbean, Mona, Jamaica, April 19–23, 1968.

[83] Wright, C. A. "The Schistosome Life-Cycle." In *Bilharziasis: International Academy of Pathology.* Edited by F. K. Mostofi. New York: Springer-Verlag, 1967. Pp. 3–7.

DIAGNOSTIC METHODOLOGY

[84] Alves, William, and Dyson M. Blair. "Diagnosis of Schistosomiasis: Intradermal Tests Using Cercarial Antigens." *Lancet* 251 (October 1946): 556–560.

[85] Bell, D. R. "A New Method for Counting *Schistosoma mansoni* Eggs in Faeces." *Bulletin of W.H.O.* 29 (1963): 525–530.

[86] Farooq, M., S. A. Samaan, and J. Nielsen. "Assessment of Severity of Disease Caused by *Schistosoma haematobium* and *S. mansoni* in the Egypt-49 Project Area." *Bulletin of W.H.O.* 35 (1966): 389–404.

[87] Faust, E. C. "The Identification and Differential Diagnosis of Helminth Parasites, Their Eggs and Larvae." In *Human Helminthology.* Edited by E. C. Faust. Philadelphia: Lea and Febiger, 1949. Pp. 581–610.

[88] Gelfand, M. "The Clinical Demonstration of the Ova of *Schistosoma mansoni*," and "The Diagnosis of *Schistosoma mansoni.*" In *A Clinical Study of Intestinal Bilharziasis in Africa.* Edited by M. Gelfand. London: Edward Arnold Ltd., 1967. Pp. 161–181.

[89] Jordan, Peter. "Egg-Output in Bilharziasis in Relation to Epidemiology, Pathology, Treatment and Control." In *Bilharziasis: International Academy of Pathology.* Edited by F. K. Mostofi. New York: Springer-Verlag, 1967. Pp. 93–103.

[90] Kloetzel, Kurt. "Some Quantitative Aspects of Diagnosis and Epidemiology in Schistosomiasis Mansoni." *American Journal of Tropical Medicine and Hygiene* 12 (1963): 334–337.

OCCURRENCE

[91] Abdel, Azim M., and Anne Gismann. "Bilharziasis Survey in Southwestern Asia, Covering Iraq, Israel, Jordan, Lebanon, Saudi Arabia, Syria, 1950–51." *Bulletin of W.H.O.* 14 (1956): 403–456.

[92] Ayad, N. "Bilharziasis Survey in British Somaliland, Eritrea, Ethiopia, Somalia, The Sudan and Yemen." *Bulletin of W.H.O.* 14 (1956): 1–117.

[93] Charles, L. J. "Malaria in the Leeward and Windward Islands, British West Indies." *American Journal of Tropical Medicine and Hygiene* 1 (November 1952) : 946–947.

[94] Cheng, Tien-Hsi. "Schistosomiasis in Mainland China, A Review of Research and Control Programs Since 1949." *American Journal of Tropical Medicine and Hygiene* 20 (January 1971) : 26–53.

[95] "Cul-de-Sac Household Parasitological Survey." Castries: Research and Control Department, Ministry of Education and Health, Government of St. Lucia, 1967.

[96] Ferguson, Frederick F. "The Ecology of *Schistosoma* in Puerto Rico." *Bulletin of the New York Academy of Medicine* 44 (March 1968) : 231–244.

[97] Jordan, Peter. "Bilharziasis in St. Lucia: Past and Present." Unpublished paper delivered at the Thirteenth Scientific Meeting of the Standing Advisory Committee for Medical Research in the British Caribbean, Mona, Jamaica, April 19–23, 1968.

[98] Panikkar, M. K. "Bilharziasis in St. Lucia." *The Journal of Tropical Medicine and Hygiene* 64 (October 1961) : 251–255.

[99] Pesigan, T. P., et al. "Studies on *Schistosoma japonicum* Infection in the Philippines." *Bulletin of W.H.O.* 18 (1958) : 345–455.

[100] Shousha, Aly Tewfik. "Schistosomiasis: A World Problem." *Bulletin of W.H.O.* 2 (1949) : 19–30.

[101] Sturrock, Robert F. "Pre-Control Studies in St. Lucia of *Biomphalaria glabrata* and *Schistosoma mansoni*." Unpublished paper delivered at the Thirteenth Scientific Meeting of the Standing Advisory Committee for Medical Research in the British Caribbean, Mona, Jamaica, April 19–23, 1968.

[102] W.H.O. *Epidemiological and Vital Statistics Report.* Vol. 13, pt. 3. Morbidity Statistics, Bilharziasis in Various Countries, pp. 315–347. Geneva: W.H.O., 1960.

[103] W.H.O. *World Health Statistics Report.* Vol. 22, pt. 2. Special Subjects, 3. Schistosomiasis, pp. 233–247. Geneva: W.H.O., 1969.

[104] Webbe, G., and P. Jordan. "Recent Advances in Knowledge of Schistosomiasis in East Africa." *Transactions of the Royal Society of Tropical Medicine and Hygiene* 60 (1966) : 279–306.

[105] Wright, W. H. "Bilharziasis as a Public Health Problem in the Pacific." *Bulletin of W.H.O.* 2 (1949) : 581–595.

[106] Wright, W. H. "Schistosomiasis as a World Problem." *Bulletin of the New York Academy of Medicine* 44 (1968) : 301–312.

PREVENTION AND CONTROL

[107] Farooq, M. "Pre-Control Investigations in Bilharziasis." *The Journal of Tropical Medicine and Hygiene* 72 (1969) : 14–18.

[108] Farooq, M. "Progress in Bilharziasis Control, The Situation in Egypt." *W.H.O. Chronicle* 21 (1967) : 175–184.

[109] Haefner, Don P., et al. "Preventive Actions in Dental Disease, Tuber-

culosis, and Cancer." *Public Health Reports* 82 (May 1967): 451–459.

[110] Hairston, Nelson G., and Benjamin C. Santos. "Ecological Control of the Snail Host of *Schistosoma japonicum* in the Philippines." *Bulletin of W.H.O.* 25 (1961): 603–610.

[111] Jordan, Peter. "Chemotherapy of Schistosomiasis." *Bulletin of the New York Academy of Medicine* 44 (1968): 245–258.

[112] Lees, Ronald E. M. "Trial of an Enteric-Coated Preparation of Lucanthone Hydrochloride in *Schistosoma mansoni* Infection." *Transactions of the Royal Society of Tropical Medicine and Hygiene* 61 (1967): 806–811.

[113] Macdonald, George. "The Dynamics of Helminth Infections, with Special Reference to Schistosomiasis." *Transactions of the Royal Society of Tropical Medicine and Hygiene* 59 (1965): 489–506.

[114] Malek, Emile A. "Bilharziasis Control in Pump Schemes near Khartoum, Sudan, and an Evaluation of the Efficacy of Chemical and Mechanical Barriers." *Bulletin of W.H.O.* 27 (1962): 41–58.

[115] McMullen, Donald B. "The Modification of Habits in the Control of Bilharziasis, with Special Reference to Water Resource Development." In *Ciba Foundation Symposium: Bilharziasis*. Edited by G. E. W. Wolstenholme and M. O'Connor. Boston: Little, Brown and Co., 1962. Pp. 382–396.

[116] McMullen, Donald B., et al. "Bilharziasis Control in Relation to Water Resources Development in Africa and the Middle East." *Bulletin of W.H.O.* 27 (1962): 25–40.

[117] Paulini, Ernest. "Bilharziasis Control by Application of Molluscicides: A Review of Its Present Status." *Bulletin of W.H.O.* 18 (1958): 975–988.

[118] Pesigan, T. P., and Nelson G. Hairston. "The Effect of Snail Control on the Prevalence of *Schistosoma japonicum* Infection in the Philippines." *Bulletin of W.H.O.* 25 (1961): 479–482.

[119] Research and Control Department, Ministry of Education and Health, Castries, St. Lucia, W.I. "Research and Control Department First Report: April, 1965–September, 1967." Mimeographed.

[120] Research and Control Department, Ministry of Education and Health, Castries, St. Lucia, W.I. "Research and Control Department Second Report: September, 1967–January, 1969." Mimeographed.

[121] Smithers, S. R. "Acquired Resistance to Bilharziasis." In *Ciba Foundation Symposium: Bilharziasis*. Edited by G. E. W. Wolstenholme and M. O'Conner. Boston: Little, Brown and Co., 1962. Pp. 36–62.

[122] Sturrock, R. F. "The Development of Irrigation and Its Influence on the Transmission of Bilharziasis in Tanganyika." *Bulletin of W.H.O.* 22 (1965): 225–236.

[123] von Ezdorf, R. H. "Demonstrations of Malaria Control." *Public Health Reports* 31 (1916): 614–629.

[124] White, Gilbert F., David J. Bradley, and Anne U. White. *Drawers of*

Water: Domestic Water Use in East Africa. Chicago: The University of Chicago Press, 1972.

[125]   W.H.O. *Chemotherapy of Bilharziasis: Report of a W.H.O. Scientific Group.* W.H.O. Technical Report Series, no. 317. Geneva: W.H.O., 1966.

[126]   W.H.O. "The Influence of Community Water Supply Programmes on Health and Social Progress." *W.H.O. Chronicle* 18 (1964): 180–191.

[127]   W.H.O. *Epidemiology and Control of Schistosomiasis: Report of a W.H.O. Expert Committee.* W.H.O. Technical Report Series, no. 372. Geneva: W.H.O., 1967.

[128]   Wright, C. A. "Some Views on Biological Control of Trematode Diseases." *Transactions of the Royal Society of Tropical Medicine and Hygiene* 62 (1968): 320–329.

ECONOMIC, SOCIAL, AND PUBLIC HEALTH ASPECTS

[129]   Andreano, Ralph L. "Schistosomiasis in the People's Republic of China: Some Public Health and Economic Aspects." The University of Wisconsin Health Economics Research Center, Madison, Wis., Research Report Series, no. 3, May 1972. Mimeographed.

[130]   Ashford, Bailey K., and Pedro Gutierrez. *Ucinariasis in Puerto Rico: A Medical and Economic Problem.* 61st Cong., 3d sess., Senate Document 808. Washington, D.C.: U.S. Government Printing Office, 1911.

[131]   Barnes, Seymour. "Malaria Eradication in Surinam: Prospects of Success After Five Years of Health Education." *International Journal of Health Education* 11 (January–March 1968): 20–31.

[132]   Bey, M. K. "The National Campaign for the Treatment and Control of Bilharziasis from the Scientific and Economic Aspects." *Journal of the Royal Egyptian Medical Association* 32 (November–December 1949): 819.

[133]   "Bilharziasis as a Man-Made Disease." *W.H.O. Chronicle* 13 (January 1959): 19–24.

[134]   Bruijning, C. F. A. "Bilharziasis in Irrigation Schemes in Ethiopia." *Tropical and Geographical Medicine* 21 (March 1969): 280–292.

[135]   Cummings, J. C., and J. H. White. "Control of Hookworm Infection at the Deep Gold Mines of Mother Loade, California." *Bureau of Mines Bulletin* 139 (1923): 1–52.

[136]   Cummins, G. "Economic Implications of Schistosomiasis." Unpublished paper delivered at Tulane University Symposium, "The Future of Schistosomiasis Control," New Orleans, La., February 1972. Mimeographed.

[137]   Farooq, M. "Medical and Economic Importance of Schistosomiasis." *The Journal of Tropical Medicine and Hygiene* 67 (May 1964): 105–112.

[138]   Farooq, M. "A Possible Approach to the Evaluation of the Economic

Burden Imposed on a Community by Schistosomiasis." *Annals of Tropical Medicine and Parasitology* 57 (September 1963): 325–331.

[139] Farooq, M., et al. "The Epidemiology of *Schistosoma haematobium* and *S. mansoni* Infections in the Egypt-49 Project Area. Part 2: Prevalence of Bilharziasis in Relation to Personal Attributes and Habits." *Bulletin of W.H.O.* 35 (1966): 293–318.

[140] Forsyth, D. M., and D. J. Bradley. "The Consequences of Bilharziasis: Medical and Public Health Importance in Northwest Tanzania." *Bulletin of W.H.O.* 34 (1966): 715–735.

[141] Foster, R. "Schistosomiasis on an Irrigated Estate in E. Africa. 3. Effects of Asymptomatic Infection on Health and Industrial Efficiency." *The Journal of Tropical Medicine and Hygiene* 70 (August 1967): 185–195.

[142] Caud, J. "The Role of Human Geography and Social Activities of Diverse Groups in a Community in the Epidemiology of Bilharziasis." *Bulletin of W.H.O.* 18 (1958): 1081–1087.

[143] Jordan, P. "Schistosomiasis and the Community." Unpublished paper delivered at Tulane University Symposium, "The Future of Schistosomiasis Control," New Orleans, La., February 1972. Mimeographed. The St. Lucian schistosomiasis mortality data, given here, are from Ronald E. M. Lees.

[144] Jordan, Peter, and Kae Randall. "Bilharziasis in Tanganyika: Observations on Its Effects and the Effects of Treatment in Schoolchildren." *The Journal of Tropical Medicine and Hygiene* 65 (January 1962): 1–6.

[145] Kieser, J. A. "Schistosomiasis: An Educational Problem." *South African Medical Journal* 21 (November 1947): 854–855.

[146] Kloetzel, K. "Mortality in Chronic Splenomegaly Due to *Schistosomiasis mansoni:* Follow-up Study in a Brazilian Population." *Transactions of the Royal Society of Tropical Medicine and Hygiene* 61 (1967): 803–805.

[147] Lanoix, Joseph N. "Relation Between Irrigation Engineering and Bilharziasis." *Bulletin of W.H.O.* 28 (1958): 1011–1035.

[148] Loveridge, F. G., W. F. Ross, and D. M. Blair. "Schistosomiasis: The Effect of the Disease on Educational Attainment." *South African Medical Journal* 22 (April 1948): 260–263.

[149] MacDonald, George. "The Assessment of the Importance of Bilharziasis." W.H.O. Symposium on Bilharziasis, Geneva, April 1960. Mimeographed. P. 17.

[150] Mousa, A. H. "Bilharziasis as a National Health Problem in the United Arab Republic." In *Ciba Foundation Symposium: Bilharziasis.* Edited by G. E. W. Wolstenholme and M. O'Conner. Boston: Little, Brown and Co., 1962. Pp. 1–6.

[151] Nabawy, M., M. Gabr, and Mohamed M. Ragab. "Effects of Bilharzia-

sis on Development of Egyptian Children." *The Journal of Tropical Medicine and Hygiene* 64 (November 1961): 271–277.

[152]   Paulini, Ernest. "Control Programmes and Socio-Economical Development." Unpublished paper, Universidade de Minas Gerais, Escola de Engenharia, Belo Horizonte, Brazil, May 1972. Typewritten.

[153]   Usborne, Vivian. "Some Notes on Urinary Bilharziasis in Sukuma School Children Especially as Regards Scholastic Performance." *The East African Medical Journal* 31 (October 1954): 451–458.

[154]   van der Schalie, Henry. "Egypt's New High Dam—Asset or Liability." *The Biologist* 42 (June 1960): 63–70.

[155]   van der Schalie, Henry. "People and Their Snail-Borne Diseases." *Michigan Quarterly Review* 2 (April 1963): 106–114.

[156]   W.H.O. *Measurement of the Public Health Importance of Schistosomiasis: Report of a W.H.O. Scientific Group*, Technical Report Series, no. 349. Geneva: W.H.O., 1967. Pp. 3–93.

[157]   Watson, J. R. "Schistosomiasis in the Tigris-Euphrates Valley with Special Reference to Its Economic Consequences." *Proceedings of the Sixth International Congress of Tropical Medicine and Malaria* 2 (1959): 203–210.

[158]   "Ways of Treating Many of the Major Diseases—Simply and Effectively—Have Yet to be Found." *The Johns Hopkins Magazine,* Summer 1967, p. 9.

[159]   Wright, Willard H. "Medical Parasitology in a Changing World. What of the Future?" *The Journal of Parasitology* 37 (February 1951): 2.

St. Lucia and the West Indies

[160]   Abbott, George C. "The West Indian Sugar Industry with Some Long-Term Projections of Supply to 1975." *Social and Economic Studies* 13, no. 1 (March 1964): 19.

[161]   Andreano, Ralph L. "Economic Development of St. Lucia." Unpublished manuscript, August 1970. Mimeographed. Available from the author, University of Wisconsin, Madison, Wis.

[162]   Breen, Henry Hegart. *St. Lucia: Historical, Statistical and Descriptive.* London: Longmans, Brown, Green and Longmans, 1844.

[163]   *Budget Address by the Honourable John G. M. Compton, Premier and Minister of Finance on the 30th December.* Castries: n.p., 1971.

[164]   Crowley, Daniel J. "Conservatism and Change in Saint Lucia." Separata del II Tomo de Actas del XXXIII Congreso Internacional de Americanistas, Celebrado en San José de Costa Rica del 20 al 27 Julio de 1958, Impreso per la Editorial Lehmann.

[165]   Crowley, Daniel J. "Naming Customs in St. Lucia." *Social and Economic Studies* 5 (March 1956): 87–92.

[166]   Cumper, G. E., ed. *The Economy of the West Indies.* Kingston: United Printers, 1960. Especially pp. 95–125.

[167] Davison, Robert Barry. *West Indian Migrants: Social and Economic Facts of Migration from the West Indies.* London: Oxford University Press, 1962.

[168] Fonaroff, L. S. "Man and Malaria in Trinidad: Ecological Perspectives of a Changing Health Hazard." *Association of American Geographers Annual* 63 (September 1968): pp. 526–556.

[169] Glick, Leonard B. "Notes on St. Lucia: A Report to the Rockefeller Foundation." Unpublished manuscript, 1969. Mimeographed. Available from the author, Hampshire College, Amherst, Mass.

[170] Glick, Leonard, and Nanci Glick. "The Working People of St. Lucia: Social, Political, and Cultural Perspectives." Unpublished manuscript, 1969, p. 108. Mimeographed. Available from the author, Hampshire College, Amherst, Mass.

[171] Guerra, Francisco. "The Influence of Disease on Race, Logistics and Colonization in the Antilles." *The Journal of Tropical Medicine and Hygiene* 69 (February 1966): 23–35.

[172] Jesse, C. *Outlines of St. Lucia's History.* 2d ed. Castries: Voice Publishing Co., 1964. Pp. 16–31.

[173] Levacher, Michael Gabriel. *Medical Guide of the Antilles.* 3d ed. Paris: Levacher, 1847.

[174] MacKenzie, Alasdair F., et al. "MacKenzie Commission of Enquiry into the Sugar Industry of St. Lucia, 1960." Health Economics Research Center, University of Wisconsin, Madison, Wis. Xeroxed.

[175] O'Loughlin, Carleen. *Economic and Political Change in the Leeward and Windward Islands.* New Haven: Yale University Press, 1968.

[176] O'Neale, H. W. "The Economy of St. Lucia." *Social and Economic Studies* 13 (December 1964): 440–470.

[177] Persaud, Bishnodat. "Some Preliminary Considerations on the Implications for the Banana Industry of the U.K. Joining the European Common Market." University of the West Indies, Institute of Social and Economic Research, Barbados, n.d. Mimeographed.

[178] Persaud, Bishnodat, et al. "Enquiry into the Feasibility of Reintroducing the Sugar Industry in St. Lucia." University of the West Indies, Eastern Caribbean, Bridgetown, Barbados, 1966. Mimeographed.

[179] Reubens, Edwin P. "Migration and Development in the West Indies." *Studies in Federal Economics.* No. 3, Jamaica, 1960. Pp. 2–6.

[180] The St. Lucia Banana Growers Association Limited. *Thirteenth Annual Ordinary General Meeting, July 9th 1966.* Castries: The Voice Publishing Company, Ltd., n.d. P. 6.

[181] St. Lucia Government. *Factsheet on St. Lucia. West Indies.* Castries: Government Printing Office, 1965. Pp. 3–6.

[182] St. Lucia Government. *Overseas Trade of St. Lucia: 1960, 1965,* and *1966.* Castries: Government Printing Office, 1964, 1967, 1969.

[183] St. Lucia Government. *Report of Customs and Excise Department for 1951.* Castries: Government Printing Office, 1953. Table 6, p. 10.

[184] St. Lucia Government. *Report of the Medical Department, 1949.* Castries: Government Printing Office, 1951.

[185] St. Lucia Government. *Report of the Medical Department, 1950.* Castries: Government Printing Office, 1952.

[186] St. Lucia Government. *Report of the Registrar of Civil Status, 1955, 1957, 1958, 1959, 1960, 1961, 1962.* Castries: Government Printing Office, 1956–1963.

[187] *St. Lucia Population Census, 1960.* Port of Spain, Trinidad: The Population Census Division, The Central Statistical Office, 1967.

[188] Shurcliff, Alice W., and John F. Wellemeyer. *Economic Development in the Eastern Caribbean Islands: St. Lucia.* Series 4: Manpower Surveys. Bridgetown, Barbadoes: University of the West Indies, Institute for Social and Economic Research, 1967.

[189] *West Indies and Caribbean Yearbook, 1970* and *1971.* Croydon, England: Thomas Skinner & Co., 1969–1970.

Sociology

[190] Abrahamson, Stephen. "Our Status System and Scholastic Rewards." *Journal of Educational Sociology* 25 (1952): 441–50.

[191] Buck, A. A., et al. *Health and Disease in Four Peruvian Villages.* Baltimore: Johns Hopkins Press, 1968.

[192] Daniels, Cora Linn, and C. M. Stevens, eds. *Encyclopedia of Superstitions, Folklore, and the Occult Sciences of the World.* Chicago: J. H. Yewdale & Sons, 1903. 3: 1431.

[193] Davie, James S. "Social Class Factors and School Attendance." *Harvard Educational Review* 23 (1953): 175–185.

[194] Douglas, J. W. B. *The Home and the School.* London: MacGibbon and Kee, 1964.

[195] Duff, R. S., and A. Hollingshead. *Sickness and Society.* New York: Harper & Row, 1968.

[196] Epstein, Erwin H. "The Absence of Observed Disease Effects on Productivity: A Socio-Cultural Explanation." Unpublished manuscript, December 1969. Mimeographed. Available from the author, Kearney State College, Kearney, Nebraska.

[197] Etzioni, Amitai. *Modern Organizations.* Englewood Cliffs, N.J.: Prentice-Hall, 1964.

[198] Evans, A. J. "The ILA V.D. Campaign." *The Rhodes-Livingstone Journal* 9 (1950): 40–47.

[199] Floud, J., and A. H. Halsey. "English Secondary Schools and the Supply of Labor." In *Education, Economy and Society.* Edited by A. H. Halsey et al. New York: The Free Press, 1961.

[200] Foster, George M. *Tzintzuntzan: Mexican Peasants in a Changing World.* Boston: Little, Brown, and Co., 1967. Pp. 123–124.

[201] Graham, Saxon. "Social Factors in Relation to Chronic Illness." In *Handbook of Medical Sociology.* Edited by Howard Freeman, Sol

Levine, and Leo G. Reeder. Englewood Cliffs, N.J.: Prentice-Hall, 1963. Pp. 65–98.

[202] Havighurst, Robert J., and Bernice L. Neugarten. "Social Structure in America." In *Society and Education*. 3d ed. Boston: Allyn and Bacon, 1967.

[203] Havighurst, Robert J., et al. *Growing Up in River City*. New York: John Wiley, 1962.

[204] Herriott, Robert E., and Nancy Hoyt St. John. *Social Class and the Urban School*. New York: John Wiley, 1966.

[205] Hollingshead, August Belmont. *Elmtown's Youth*. New York: John Wiley, 1949.

[206] Homans, George Caspar. *The Human Group*. New York: Harcourt, Brace & Co., 1950.

[207] Husen, Torsten, et al., eds. *International Study of Achievement in Mathematics: A Comparison of Twelve Countries*. New York: John Wiley, 1967.

[208] Koos, Earl Loman. *The Health of Regionville: What the People Thought and Did About It*. New York: Hafner Publishing Co., 1954.

[209] Lewis, Oscar. *La Vida: A Puerto Rican Family in the Culture of Poverty*. New York: Vintage Books, 1968.

[210] Lewis, Oscar. "Medicine and Politics in a Mexican Village." In *Health, Culture and Community: Case Studies of Public Relations to Health Programs*. Edited by Benjamin D. Paul. New York: Russell Sage Foundation, 1955. Pp. 429–430.

[211] Lowell, Anthony M. *Socio-Economic Conditions and Tuberculosis Prevalence in New York City, 1949–51*. New York: New York Tuberculosis and Health Association, 1956.

[212] Machlachlan, John M. "Cultural Factors in Health and Disease." In *Patients, Physicians, and Illness: Sourcebook in Behavioral Science and Medicine*. Edited by E. Gartly Jaco. New York: The Free Press, 1958. Pp. 95–96.

[213] Marriot, McKim. "Western Medicine in a Village of Northern India." In *Health, Culture and Community: Case Studies of Public Relations to Health Programs*. Edited by Benjamin D. Paul. New York: Russell Sage Foundation, 1955. P. 239.

[214] Middleton, Russell, and Charles M. Grigg. "Rural-Urban Differences in Aspirations." *Rural Sociology* 24 (December 1959): 347–354.

[215] Miner, Horace. "Culture Under Pressure: A Hausa Case." *Human Organization* 19, no. 3 (Fall, 1960): 164–167.

[216] Nelson, M. J. *The Nelson Reading Test, Grades 3–9*. Boston: Houghton Mifflin, 1962.

[217] Pavlid, Vasile. "Research into the Health Knowledge and Behavior of School Children." *International Journal of Health Education* 11 (1968): 118–119.

[218] Piaget, Jean. *The Child's Conception of Number*. Translated by

C. Geottegno and F. M. Hodgson. London: Routledge and Kegan Paul, 1952.

[219] Piaget, Jean, and Barbel Inhelder. *The Growth of Logical Thinking from Childhood to Adolescence.* Translated by Anne Parsons and Stanley Milgram. New York: Basic Books, 1958.

[220] Richardson, Alan, and John Woolcott. "A Social Survey of Community Attitudes to Cancer." *International Journal of Health Education* 10 (July–September, 1967): 143.

[221] Roethlisberger, Fritz Jules, and William J. Dickson. *Management and the Worker.* Cambridge: Harvard University Press, 1939. P. 572.

[222] Saunders, Lyle. "Healing Ways in the Spanish Southwest." In *Patients, Physicians, and Illness: Sourcebook in Behavioral Science and Medicine.* Edited by E. Gartly Jaco. New York: The Free Press, 1958. Pp. 234–255.

[223] Sewell, William H., Archie O. Haller, and Murray A. Straus. "Social Status and Educational and Occupational Aspiration." *American Sociological Review* 22 (1957): 67–73.

[224] Sexton, Thomas. "Analysis of a Communicational Breakdown in the Surinam Malaria Eradication Programme." *International Journal of Health Education* 9 (July–September, 1966): 124–126.

[225] Shaw, Duane C. "The Relation of Socio-Economic Status to Educational Achievement in Grades Four to Eight." *Journal of Educational Research* 37 (1943): 197–201.

[226] Stephenson, Richard M. "Mobility Orientation and Stratification of 1,000 Ninth Graders." *American Sociological Review* 22 (1957): 204–212.

[227] Terman, L. M., et al. *Mental and Physical Traits of a Thousand Gifted Children.* Stanford: Stanford University Press, 1925.

[228] Whiteman, J. "Social Factors Influencing Health Education Among the Chimbu." *International Journal of Health Education* 9 (January–March, 1966): 12.

[229] Whiting, John W. M., and Irvin L. Child. *Child Training and Personality: A Cross-Cultural Study.* New Haven: Yale University Press, 1953.

[230] Whyte, William Forte, et al. *Money and Motivation.* New York: Harper, 1955.

[231] Zborowsky, Mark. "Cultural Components of Responses to Pain." *Journal of Social Issues* 8 (1952): 16–30.

Miscellaneous

[232] Ackerknecht, Erwin H. "The Role of Medical History in Medical Education." *Bulletin of the History of Medicine* 21 (March–April, 1947): 135–145.

[233] Hirsch, August. *Handbook of Geographical and Historical Pathology.* Translated from the 2d ed. by Charles Creighton. 3 vols. London: The New Sydenham Society, 1883–1886. 1: 220, 382, 635–639; 2: 34, 195, 304–305; 3: 28–29, 106.

[234] Jordan, Peter. Correspondence. December 8, 1969. Available from Burton A. Weisbrod, University of Wisconsin, Madison, Wis.

[235] Jordan, Peter. Correspondence. May 13, 1969. Available from Erwin H. Epstein, Kearney State College, Kearney, Nebraska.

[236] Malthus, Thomas R. *An Essay on the Principles of Population.* 6th ed. London: John Murray, 1826. 1: 514, 522–527.

[237] McKeown, Thomas. "Medicine and World Population." A Symposium on Research Issues in Public Health and Population Change held at the Graduate School of Public Health, University of Pittsburgh, Pittsburgh, Pa., June 1964. Mimeographed.

[238] Myrdal, Gunnar. *The Asian Drama.* New York: Pantheon, 1968. Especially 3: 1616–1617.

[239] U.N., ILO, and UNESCO. "Report on International Definition and Measurement of Standards and Levels of Living." Committee of Experts Reports, E/CN, 179, W.H.O., Geneva, 1954. P. 321.

INDEX

Academic impact of disease. *See* Scholastic impact of disease

Age: and births, 109; and deaths, 111–112; and parasite prevalence, 114–115, 171; productivity effect of, 141; and sample bias, 171–173, 178–181

Ascaris, 54–55, 61, 85; natality impact of, 66; effect on rural labor productivity of, 74n; effect on urban labor productivity of, 76; pooled quantitative findings on, 79–80

Aswan High Dam: and schistosomiasis increase, 55, 188

Auster, Richard, 110n

Babonneau school. *See* Scholastic impact of disease

Backward-bending labor supply, 184, 186

Barlow, Robin, 22–23

Bayluscide: as snail-eradication compound, 51

Bell, D. R., 63n

Benefit-cost framework: definitional problems and, 4; and resource allocation for disease control, 5; and spillover effects of health outlays, 7, 67; and human life valuation, 8; and public expenditure theory, 21; for alternative control methods, 21; limited utilization in LDCs of, 24; relative to schistosomiasis, 56

Bernoulli, J., 13

Budgetary behavior: relevance of, 60, 82

Causality direction problem, 23–24, 83–84; in natality analysis, 65, 105–107; in work attendance, 75; in scholastic analysis, 124–125, 129–130; in labor productivity analysis, 138–139; between development and disease, 188; between schistosomiasis and banana cultivation, 191

Chadwick, Edwin, 9, 15, 17, 18

Clearkin, P. A., 53

Cul-de-Sac Valley: population characteristics in, 168. *See also* Labor productivity impact of disease, rural; Natality impact of disease; Survey data

Debilitation: as change in relative prices, 72; of spirit as constraint, 87, 88

Debility and disability measurement: handled by Fisher, 20

DESIGNED BY
SYLVIA SOLOCHEK WALTERS
MANUFACTURED BY KINGSPORT PRESS, INC., KINGSPORT, TENNESSEE
TEXT LINES ARE SET IN BODONI BOOK, DISPLAY LINES
IN BASKERVILLE AND BODONI BOOK

Ⓤ

Library of Congress Cataloging in Publication Data
Main entry under title:
Disease and economic development.
Bibliography: p. 197–213.
1. Hygiene, Public—St. Lucia—Statistics.
2. Medical parasitology—Statistics. 3. St. Lucia—
Social conditions. 4. St. Lucia—Economic conditions.
I. Weisbrod, Burton Allen, 1931—
RA456.S25D57   338.01   72–7997
ISBN 0–299–06340–2